A Stroke in the Family

Valerie Eaton Griffith

Edited by David Worsley,
with revised Preface and additional Forewords

First published in Great Britain 1970
by Penguin Books Ltd.
Published in 1975 by Wildwood House Limited.
Reprinted 1979, 1986

Published in 2010 by East Kent Strokes,
with help from a community grant from
J.S. Sainbury's (Canterbury store)

Cover design by Green & Tempest

Printed and bound in Great Britain by
CPI Antony Rowe, Chippenham and Eastbourne

ISBN   978-0-9565126-0-4

Contents

Preface by Dr. Anthony Rudd

I am very honoured to be asked to write a preface to this unique book. There are very few books available that provide practical information for stroke survivors and their carers. This short book manages to provide clear sensible advice on how to help someone with communication problems as well as conveying a real sense of optimism that is unfortunately so often lacking from health professionals.

When I first started as a consultant physician at St. Thomas' Hospital in London over 20 years ago the medical treatment of stroke was regarded as something that required no specialist skills. Often the decision would be made by the General Practitioner to keep a patient at home because there was nothing to be gained by admitting them to hospital. If they were admitted very little active treatment would be offered unless they were admitted to the geriatric ward where there was some rudimentary rehabilitation.

Stroke care has changed dramatically in the last decade. It has been shown that people looked after on a specialist stroke unit are much more likely to recover than those cared for on a general ward. Nearly everyone now has a brain scan which is something I literally had to fight for in the early years; indeed the only time I have been hit by a fellow consultant was when I was trying to persuade a radiologist that a particular patient needed a scan. We now have access to clot busting treatment that can cure some people who would otherwise have a severe disabling stroke and research has shown that rehabilitation can be effective with a clear link between the amount someone receives and the outcome.

However, the one thing that most stroke sufferers complain about is that they do not receive enough treatment and that is certainly the case in the majority of UK hospitals. If the situation is inadequate in hospital then it is even worse once the person gets home. We are attempting to improve community rehabilitation but still too often there are long waiting lists and then woefully infrequent treatment sessions that stop too soon. The amount of treatment that Pat received in a week using the system described in this book probably equates to the total amount received by the average stroke patient in the UK in a year.

There is no such thing as a typical stroke patient. The first thing I teach all the doctors, nurses and therapists who work with me, is that everyone needs to be treated as an individual. The extent of the damage to the brain as a result of the stroke will vary and their previous skills, interests and personality all need to be understood when planning and delivering treatment. The second thing they need to learn is something that is highlighted in this book, which is that recovery can go on for a long time and anyone who thinks that all the recovery is going to take place within the first three months or even three years is mistaken.

Perhaps the most important message that I have taken from this book is that we should not be relying on professional therapists to provide all the treatment that is needed. It is feasible for 'amateurs' to contribute an enormous amount and hopefully this book will give such people the confidence to help.

One useful analogy is the person attempting to learn how to play the piano, a skill requiring development of new connections and pathways within the brain. If they relied completely on the lessons given weekly without regular practice in between, little if any progress would be made. The brain adapts only with frequent and often repetitive practice. The same processes are taking place within the brain when a stroke patient is relearning lost skills such as balance, walking and communication. The parent of the child learning the piano often provides the crucial role of encouraging, persuading and sometimes gentle bullying that Valerie provided to Pat and Alan.

Please read this book if you know anyone who has had a stroke. I hope it will inspire you to do what Valerie did and in so doing make a real difference to their life

Dr. Anthony Rudd
Stroke Physician Guy's and St. Thomas' Hospital,
and Clinical Director for Stroke in London

Roald Dahl's Foreword

When Pat came out of hospital in California, she received professional speech therapy for one hour a day for four weeks. This was a beginning. But it was easy to see that it was not going to be enough. By the time she arrived home in England, she was still about seventy five per cent aphasic. She could neither read, write nor handle numbers. She had no initiative. If left alone, she would sit and stare into space and in half an hour a great black cloud of depression would envelop her mind. Unless I was prepared to have a bad tempered desperately unhappy nitwit in the house, some very drastic action would have to be taken at once. Pat, I decided, must be kept occupied, at any rate in the early stages, for at least six hours a day. I made this decision the day after we got home. I called in no doctors. It was a matter that had to be resolved entirely by the family.

A couple of days later I had managed to initiate a crash programme of amateur teaching. This was not difficult to do. I simply telephoned as many female relatives and friends as I could think of and asked them for an hour or two of their time each week. I made a roster or timetable and stuck it on the kitchen wall. The first lesson was to be at nine, the second at ten and the third at eleven. At noon Pat would knock off for lunch and then take a nap. At two p.m. the fourth teacher of the day would arrive, followed by another at 3 p.m. and another at 4 p.m. And so the lessons began. The teachers arrived punctually. They never let me down. For six hours a day, five days a week, these remarkable and persistent people came trooping into the house. I myself took no part in these lessons, except to settle each new teacher in on her first day and to calm her nervousness and make suggestions as to how to proceed. 'Good heavens,' they would say to me as they arrived at the door the first time. 'I don't know a thing about it. What on earth shall I do with her? I'm not a speech therapist.' And so on. But after they had overcome their initial trepidation, not a single one of our fifteen teachers needed any further instruction. They seemed to know instinctively just what to do with Pat, when to put the pressure on, when to play games, when to relax and take a walk in the garden. And with this system going smoothly, I myself was left more or less free to do some work and to run the house and to organize the children.

After about six months of this really tough routine, Pat had had enough. She wanted a rest. So I began slowly to reduce the number of lessons each day. But these splendid amateur teachers had in that time lifted the patient's intellectual ability by roughly another twenty five per cent. So she was now about halfway back to complete recovery.

It was at this point that Val Eaton Griffith slipped quietly into her life and took over. Instead of the tough daily grind of several lessons from several different people (something that I think was absolutely essential in the first place), Val gave her a couple of hours each morning and homework to do later on in the day when she felt like it. For nearly two years this routine went on. Slowly, insidiously and quite relentlessly, Val coaxed her back to where she is now - virtually one hundred per cent recovered.

Nothing, mind you, could have been accomplished without Pat's extraordinary guts. Nor in my opinion without the six months of really hard work by her fifteen teachers in the first place. But the fact remains that Val's performance was of the very highest order. The more I think of it, the more I begin to doubt whether anyone else could have accomplished it. Without any medical knowledge whatsoever, Val has now become a genuine expert in the mental rehabilitation of brain injured persons.

Her methods are quite simple to follow, but they were not simple to evolve. Very few people have much of an idea of what to do when faced with a brain injured friend or relative. I know this to be true because 1 have read every one of the thousands and thousands of letters that have poured into our house during the last four years. Every one of them is a cry for help.

Val is a modest lady. It wasn't her idea to write this book. In fact, it wasn't until we showed her just one crate full of these 'stroke patient letters' that we were able to persuade her to put her methods down on paper.

Here they are. Do not be deceived by their simplicity, for therein lies the secret of their success. They work. I can guarantee that. Everyone who has a stroke patient in the family should have this little book at hand. It is a manual for the families and friends of all stroke patients everywhere.

But to go back for a moment to the beginning. A few weeks after Pat had had her stroke and she was able to travel, we set out for Los Angeles airport to catch a plane to England. At the airport we were met by about fifty reporters and cameramen and were compelled to hold a sort of press-conference. It was a crazy affair because Pat was not only crippled but was unable to answer any of their questions except in monosyllables. When I told them that one day she would act again, the room became silent. The reporters stared. I might just as well have announced that the woman was going to sprout wings and fly to the moon. I'm not sure, mind you, that I believed what I said. But it was vital to make Pat believe it. She had to have a powerful incentive and this was it. So throughout the months and months of hard slogging that were to follow, I never stopped telling her that she would one day go back to work. I told her so often that she began to believe it herself and that was a victory.

After every great effort comes the moment of truth. Pat's moment came after she had been working for two years with Val. It was a request from the Association for Brain Injured Children in New York that she make the major speech at a huge seventy five-dollar-a-ticket dinner to raise funds for the Society. In fact they would like to build the entire show around Pat, calling it 'An Evening with Patricia Neal'. Pat said, 'No, I can't do it.' I said. 'You've got to.' She said, 'Will you come with me?' I said, 'No. You're on your own now.' In the end, very reluctantly, she agreed to go provided Val went along as well and introduced her from the platform. Speeches were written, one for Val and one for Pat. Rehearsals began. And now suddenly, a magic thing began to happen. Pat realized that she was going to have to give a public performance. The old pro smelled the smell of battle once again and she sprang to life. She rehearsed her speech with almost as much vigour as she would have rehearsed a Broadway play. Then she and Val flew over and the great night arrived. Fourteen hundred people, most of them folk of considerable consequence, filled the ballroom of the Waldorf-Astoria. Val, trembling greatly, made a brave and modest introductory speech. Then Pat walked on to the stage and the place exploded. To these people she was back from the dead and they were cheering not only the woman herself but the immensely comforting thought that it is possible for anyone, given a lot of guts and a bit of luck, to overcome gigantic misfortunes and terrible illness. She had done it. She had proved it possible. And that meant others could do the same.

Patricia Neal's Foreword

I once acted in a play called The Miracle Worker. It was about an astonishing woman called Anne Macey but known as 'Teacher' to her pupil, Helen Keller. Miss Keller was deaf, dumb and blind, and until her Teacher exploded into her life she had nothing to live for. But from then on she learned so wonderfully to communicate with the outside world that she finally became, as you all know, a fine and famous person.

Now I would not for one moment presume to compare myself with Helen Keller. But I would most certainly presume to compare my Teacher with hers. She exploded into my life at exactly the right time. Her name is Val. She has written this book. All I can say is that if anyone has a stroke patient or a brain injured person in their family, he or she should read this book. I think it is marvellous.

Lucy Moorehead's Foreword

Alan Moorehead is a professional writer, accustomed to working eight to nine hours every day of his life, Sundays included. Four of these hours were given up to writing his books, four or five to reading, mostly research; the rest of the time he would talk with his friends.

When he came out of hospital after his illness he could not write, or read, and spoke only a few words with difficulty. Professional therapists set him on the slow way to recovery, but there still remained the problem of empty time, of hours and days which needed to be filled with some sort of constructive, hopeful work. It was a miracle of good fortune to find Val Eaton Griffith and the group of people who had worked with Pat Neal and were prepared to work with Alan, and the year he spent with them not only helped his recovery but gave us all a feeling of optimism for the future. He followed the programmes of work and the exercises described in this most practical book with concentration and devotion, and this in itself was of very great value.

No two people are alike, in sickness or in health, and some of the things that were good for Pat did not always work with Alan; Pat's is a success story which cannot easily be matched. Different methods and approaches had to be evolved and tried. But the important thing is to work; you cannot work more than a certain amount with professionals, but if you have friends who will help you, and - more important - know how to help you, then you will never give up. This book is for the friends.

Editor's Foreword

If you have made an intensive search on the internet about aphasia then you will probably have discovered that there are many forms.

Don't get confused. It has little to do with the work that you must do to help your patient.

Think just for a moment about your (assume male) patient as though he were a plant that will thrive with just three elements: sunlight; soil; and water. Now return to today and realise that he will thrive when you give him: mental stimulus; mental exercise; and repetition.

Of course, just as plants vary their needs vary. Some need full sun, others shade. Similarly, varieties of more or less water, types of soil. They also differ throughout their lives. So too will your patient's needs vary as time passes when his capacities and stamina grow.

The original text by Valerie Eaton-Griffith is a comprehensive guide to helping a stroke patient recover much from their stroke. My only edit is to hint at resources that are available today.

The carer, relative or friend who reads this in the immediate period following the stroke, will be be laden down with the shock, and an overpowering desire to understand 'Why?' and 'How can I help?' This burden, and the emotions that it brings, may cause a condition best described as 'Cannot see the wood for the trees'. It is therefore in the spirit of helping the temporarily blind that I add notes and an appendix with a guide to the resources available today - but not so 40 years ago.

I had my stroke 5 years ago and have spent 4 of these editing a newsletter for the local support group East Kent Strokes. Our experience has taught me some good news, and bad news. The good news is that almost every stroke patient will improve. The bad news is that it can take years, and will take constant and continual effort by both patient and supporter.

In one important respect, nothing has changed. The NHS still have the expertise, but not the resources to park a therapist in your home once a day for the months needed. This is why this book is so incredibly important.

Do, please, try to energise a band of volunteers to come and bring communication back into your patient's life - and his carers.

1 - Help from ordinary friends

When Patricia Neal was hit by a massive series of strokes, the surgeon, the nurses and her husband, Roald Dahl, had to fight for her life. By a miracle of skill and care she came through. After a few weeks she was home, and Roald was faced with a moment of truth.

Now all the responsibility was his - for their home and their children. And on top of this Pat was frozen by inertia, unable to help herself, unable to talk, surrounded by friends yet totally apart from them. Her world was made up of confusion, frustration, despair and boredom. She was in vital need of her husband's every minute.

Roald understood his wife's urgent need of help and her dependence on him. But he had a thousand times too much to do, Pat had a thousand times too little, and, though this doesn't sound anything very terrible, it was a killer. Physically, emotionally and mentally he was at danger point: and Pat was at the other end of the scale.

He could not shoulder all the new responsibilities and yet be permanently at Pat's side. With all the good will in the world this simply was not possible. Yet without a bottomless pit of money and great good fortune, no one can employ speech therapists for several hours a day for 500 days.

Physiotherapy was an easier problem. A twice weekly visit was wise and practicable. But it is not the physical side with which we are concerned here. It is the mental and emotional side.

It was at this point - the moment they arrived back in

21

A Stroke in the Family

England - that Roald devised the plan for Pat that is the basis of this book. He rang up the members of his family, neighbours and friends, sometimes even friends of friends, and asked if they would give one, two or three hours a week helping with Pat's rehabilitation. He worked out a schedule of visitors that kept her occupied six hours a day.

I did not know the Dahls when the whisper spread through our village of Patricia Neal's stroke. But it is the kind of bad news that leaves a shock wave of disbelief in its wake. Surely, a stroke hits only the very old? Not the warm, vibrant woman I had seen on the screen. It paralyses, doesn't it?

Then, as is the way in a village, I began to learn more. The medical profession had done wonders, but Pat was in a bad way. She could not talk. Her leg was in a brace. She was pregnant.

But this involved me only on the humanitarian level of sympathy for suffering. It never for a moment crossed my mind that I could help. How could anyone help, who knew neither Pat nor anything at all about a stroke? And - because we did not know one another - I was not one of the people Roald called.

At least, not for six months, when one of the teachers suggested me. At that point Pat's baby was born and she rebelled against returning to the old routine. But Roald was not content to let things rest. He called me, and asked if I'd work with Pat.

Who - me? Trial and Error

For a reason I don't understand the horrified 'No!'

wouldn't come from my mouth, so I said 'Yes' instead. Roald's voice was kind over the line, but I was too busy kicking myself for being the biggest fool in Christendom to take in what he said. How could I possibly help? Wouldn't I do harm instead? Why on earth had my vocabulary been reduced to yes and no? Why had yes won the day?

I tried to pull myself together and to think of something in my past life which might enable me to help. The first results were hopeless: playing tennis, walking, taking a winter holiday in order to go skiing.... The sports I had loved were no use to Pat, and they were no longer of any use to me, either. For my life, too, had been changed by illness. I could scarcely walk, and the four walls of even our happy home were too small a world.

Let me begin at the beginning.

We lived a happy family life in London. My father bore the scars of the First World War, but he had overcome his disability with courage. Then came the Second World War. I left school at 15 and worked as a Junior Civil Servant until I was 17 and old enough to join the A.T.S., the women's branch of the Army. I manned searchlights in the suburbs of London and got bombed continuously, just like everyone else. Our house was flattened, so, at the end of the war, we moved to our present home in Great Missenden, recovered a bit, and began to think of the future. Eventually, I joined Elizabeth Arden, where I worked for about ten years.

And then I was stricken with a particularly fierce kind of thyroid trouble which landed me in hospital for five months and this eventually kept me from regular work.

A Stroke in the Family

About ten years later, when I was called to help Pat, I still limped almost as badly as she did and was taking around twenty aspirins a day for the pain.

The only reason I set down these brief autobiographical details is to reassure you that nothing in my previous life in any way equipped me to deal with a stroke patient. I started from scratch, just as the reader must. It wasn't impossibly difficult, I promise you.

Such methods of teaching as I evolved were truly hit or miss. I only held hard to one thing: if anything I tried with Pat - or later, Alan - was a 'miss', I stopped it immediately and tried another approach, and another and another. Eventually you find one that works, and here is your opening.

Not one of us who worked through four years with Patricia Neal and Alan Moorehead had any qualifications whatever. We found it took a little time for us to get the feel for our task, but after several weeks we were enthusiastic and optimistic. It is the result of our practical experience with Pat and Alan that is the subject of this book, which I hope will be of help to stroke victims, their families and friends.

What you can do

Because Pat is a film star millions of people have heard her story. Since her extraordinary recovery thousands and thousands of frustrated, desperate, courageous 'next-of-kin' have written to her for help. Sometimes the patients themselves have also written, but often they cannot or do not have the will to compose a letter. Many interesting things come from these letters, but one urgent appeal rings like a prayer through every single one of them. What can we do? How can I help my husband, my wife, my son, my mother? They all contain the same question, wrung from the same despairing emptiness that is left after the doctors have gone.

This is what we suggest:

First, ring your friends and neighbours. You will be surprised how willing they will be to give up a few hours a week to helping. And second, make out a roster so that they all have their particular times and the patient's day is filled with lessons.

According to his fitness, you may find a nap in the afternoons a good idea. If so, you can arrange his schedule to include this. Say lessons from different friends at 9.30, 10.30, 11.30, then lunch and a rest, lessons again at 3 o'clock, 4 o'clock, 5 o'clock. But this, of course, you can arrange as best suits each individual case. If you cannot find enough people to fill all these hours, fill as many as you can. Or perhaps try lessons of two hours' duration.

To begin with, when teachers are nervous, let them share a lesson. Some, you may find, will continue to prefer sharing. Others will want to teach on their own.

As each new teacher volunteers, we found it helpful to invite her to sit in on a lesson in progress. This gives her some idea of what is being done and reduces her feeling of tension. The new recruit to the team is likely to be surprised at the 'professional' approach the other housewives-turned-teachers have developed. It generally takes no more than three weeks for them to become old hands, with a growing pride in their work.

Let me give you an example.

After we had been working with Pat for many months Roald asked me and the original team to meet at his house. Lucy Moorehead, he explained, was bringing Alan to visit. Alan and Lucy Moorehead had heard of Pat's illness and her remarkable progress. They wanted to learn what had been done to help. Alan, like Pat, had worked with words all his adult life, he as an author and she as an actress. This gave them something in common, other than illness. For both of them, difficulty with speaking or writing meant an end to their careers.

Lucy, Pat and Roald sat on one sofa talking hard. Alan sat on the other, around him twelve clinically minded housewives.

'How are you, Alan?' one of them asked.

'I'm very well, thank you,' he answered.

(Good, he can say these simple words perfectly. Let's stretch him a bit.)

'Where do you live, Alan?'

He points and makes gestures telling us his home is far away.

(Good, he has understood. Not so good, he could not answer in words.)

'Here are thirteen playing cards, Alan. Will you sort them in suits and seniority?'

Again, he has understood. But he only manages to sort the cards into reds and blacks, with court cards at the front. (So colours okay, pictures easily identified. Shapes and numbers not so hot. Indeed, as we subsequently discovered, at this stage Alan could identify colours only if they contrasted strongly. He found it difficult, for example, to distinguish blue from green or orange from yellow. Clearly, he did not suffer from the usual forms of colour blindness, but had a difficulty that was all his own. It will be interesting for you to discover, and work on, your patient's form of colour difficulty.)

'Add two and three, Alan.'

He holds up five fingers.

(Figures not total strangers. There may be easier recognition of the spoken than of the written word.)

'Here's a typewriter, Alan. Try typing your name.'

He finds the A, but the other letters elude him.

(Good. He can pick out one letter. Scope here.)

'What day is it, Alan?'

He searches eagerly for something to write on. (Good. He knows the answer although he cannot say it.)

From the other sofa Roald cracked a joke, heard by everyone in the room. Twelve pairs of eyes slewed secretly round to look at Alan. Had he caught the joke? He was laughing with obvious understanding.

(Good. Very good. He is aware. And he seems relaxed yet keen with all of us around him. Good again.)

At this moment Alan raised a finger and swept it slowly in an arc around him, pointing from one to the other of us. His face was passionately earnest. 'Would you -?' he said to each of us. 'Would you -?' Lucy nodded her head in support of the half phrased question, ready as always to interpret. But this time there was no need to interpret. We knew Alan was asking us if we would work with him as we had with Pat. Yes, of course we would.

'We'll rent a cottage in the village,' Lucy said. So this was when Alan's story began.

2 - Understanding the patient

The remaining chapters in this book are about working with a stroke patient, as our experience has taught us. But first there are several things that it is important to consider.

A person who has had a stroke has not reverted to a state of childhood. He is emotionally adult. He is a man without the ability to communicate. He has lessened powers of concentration. He probably has a poor memory. He is a man whose confidence may have been shattered and who is in danger of losing his self respect through no fault of his own. Never talk down to him.

He is not odd or 'touched' in the way that a lunatic is. Therefore, think of it this way: he is you or me hit by trouble and in need of help.

With a light touch

The light approach is always best. Be encouraging and laugh with him. And above all keep a businesslike, unemotional approach. This is a particularly important point for women to bear in mind - and, because men are away at work, you will probably find the majority of teachers will be women.

Take trouble to keep the patient out of the way of undue stress (however trivial or awkward making the cause appears to be). Do not shield him from the general run of 'woes'. Separate this carefully from real stress. For instance, he should be told if a child of his fails an important examination; but should this same child have a party which gets out of control, he should not be left trying to exercise authority. In the first case he will be upset, but no more than you or I. In the second case the children will almost certainly flout his stumbling efforts at authority: he will find it unbearable and may react with unreasonable force. In other words, for him to be emotional is all right. For him to be irritated beyond his ability to control himself is not.

The teacher must try to be firm, to have authority. She must have a programme for each lesson. The stroke patient will fear like the plague the person who walks in and says, 'And what shall we do now?'

Don't delay

It can be vitally important to start these lessons quickly, immediately the patient is freed by the doctors. Pat was working one month after being at death's door, one day after coming out of hospital. For her, the early days made learning and rehabilitation much easier. And getting to work straight away stemmed the tendency to sink further into apathy and despair.

In some cases it is a fact that the longer rehabilitation is delayed after brain damage has taken place, the less good the results will be. Pat started on the first day out of hospital. If she had started one year later she might have lost for ever a certain - probably a considerable - percentage of her recovery quotient. Most doctors, by the way, say that after two years no further improvement takes place. So far as Pat and Alan are concerned, this has not been true. Improvement continues, though more slowly, well beyond that point. In Pat's case, after four years, she is still improving. So, also, is Alan, after a two year period.

Lastly, get the patient out and about as much as possible. Here lies a tremendous stimulus, the need for which cannot be over stressed. Perhaps you can find one or two teachers who would be prepared to have the lessons in their homes. This means transport, but at all costs it ought to be arranged.

By getting this schedule set up you solve several pressing problems. You yourself are freer to get on with your work. You are released from some of the tensions and can more easily ensure that a happy atmosphere exists in the home. The patient is a person again, an ego. He feels he is working with purpose for his own good, his relationship with his friends is on a good footing. He is stimulated, and has an emotional outlet. His relationship with his wife, or hers with her husband, is no longer one of teacher/pupil. It is one of man and wife.

Normality, please

It is important that as many friends as possible come to see the stroke patient, and that they come as soon as possible after his illness. This will help prevent the patient from feeling in any way ostracized or 'untouchable'.

During my many years with Elizabeth Arden, I worked with makeup on many a terribly scarred face. This work did not worry me, in fact I loved it, but I learned that others found it upsetting. Some people have a fear of abnormality. A Battle of Britain pilot whose face is atrociously burned, leaving him without nose or lips, a man with a club foot or no hand, a mongol child, a stroke victim - these people can evoke a feeling of panic in others. So it is the responsibility of the wife, or whoever is in command, to encourage all the couple's friends to behave normally, to breeze in and treat the patient as if nothing had happened.

Four weeks after Pat's stroke, such film star friends as Anne Bancroft, Mildred Dunnock, Gary Grant, Margaret Leighton and Arthur Kennedy came to see her. They treated her as if she were a queen - and to this day Pat remembers their superb welcome with gratitude.

3 Re-assurance and planning

Now to get down to how these neighbours-turned-teachers can help.

The first hurdle to be cleared will probably be your anxiety about having no medical qualifications for the job. The second will almost certainly be nervousness. Together they will sum up to a string of statements and questions that may run something like this:

> You want me to help?
> But I don't know a thing about strokes!
> What can I do?
> How will I start?
> How on earth can I help?
> Are you sure you mean me?
> But what can I possibly do?

It is the purpose of this book to answer just such questions and to try to convince you that your help is of value.

When I first began working with Pat, one thing above all helped me to conquer my own personal fears. Very simply it was this: I imagined I was the one who had had a stroke, I was the one who had been so hard hit and was so desperately in need of help. This imagined reversal of roles worked an odd little miracle. There is always something of self care in our nervousness, and this flight of fancy shifted the whole emphasis away from worry about how I could possibly cope. Instead it made me think solely of Pat.

A Stroke in the Family

You may well find, as we did, that the majority of your fellow teachers will be housewives. They are obviously in a better position than most to spare an hour or two a week for the lessons.

As a housewife, then, you probably already have some experience in teaching your own children. When you come to teaching a stroke victim, some problems will remain the same but some will essentially be different. In a curious way it may well be easier, for you are an adult with the same world battered process of thought as your pupil. You do not have to look through a child's clear, fresh eyes.

The patience you will need is the same, the idea of capturing his interest and holding his elusive concentration is the same, but your standards, expectations and approach will be different. I have previously mentioned that a stroke patient has not reverted to a state of childhood, and it is vital to remember this.

Who was he?, and what can he do now?

It is good to take a moment to think of the patient as he was before the stroke. What sort of a man was he? What was his job? What were his interests? What were his strong points, his weaknesses?

Then move on as you work with him to find out what remains of his capabilities and interests. I believe you will discover that some are left complete, some are half there as it were, veiled in mist, and some have apparently gone.

Also, as you work with him, it is wise to study his frame of mind. This is not easy. To discover a man's feelings is no simple matter at the best of times, and is even harder with a stroke victim. Yet it is important for you to understand as much as possible about him so that you can work together on the same wavelength. Every one of us have a seventh veil and every one of us uses a defensive mechanism to protect his inner self. I believe that those who have been badly hurt develop this defensive mechanism to a much greater extent. And there is danger here: a danger of the teacher accepting at face value things that are not completely true.

Let me give you an example. All through the years of Pat's recovery she said she never wanted to act again. But this was not the whole truth. Pat feared that she might be unable to work again, and it was happier for her to convince herself that she did not want to work rather than face too early the possible future horror of trial and failure.

In our opinion, with a stroke patient, it is best to appear to accept their statement, yet nevertheless to continue working on the undeclared assumption that he will work again. Thus, Pat kept her sorely needed self protection and yet was strangely pleased to be actually working towards attaining a comeback in films.

Four conditions to expect

The results of strokes can cover a wide field, so it is important to take, as it were, each patient on his own merits. Patricia Neal and Alan Moorehead, for instance, had some needs and inabilities in common, but they also had many, many things that called for different approaches and different methods of teaching.

Four major things we found were essential to both, and perhaps to all stroke patients.

First, as concentration is short lived, the teacher is wise to flit from subject to subject like a bee sucking nectar, first to one flower, then to the next and the next. The stroke patient will have a better chance of summoning his reserves of concentration if he has continually a new subject to work on. He will probably fail to keep concentration on one subject, but he will succeed with something different.

Second, it is good to try to vary the actual approach, the way you go about trying to pursue any one subject. If one approach fails, try another, and another. You will suddenly hit on one narrow path which is open to the patient. Let me give you an instance of what I mean, for it is important. In the early days of working with Alan we wanted to see if he could manage the alphabet. Could he say it? No. Could he write it? No. Could he write one letter, say the letter E? No. Can he learn it by rote? No. Deadlock. The alphabet is a closed book to him. But is it? Look what happened. Alan, as a great traveller, is incredibly knowledgeable about the world. He has been everywhere and with his high intelligence is passionately interested. He could put his finger on almost any place mentioned on the globe. Then one day I said to him, 'Where is Finse, Alan?' And he had never heard of it. I turned to the index of an atlas and said, 'Find it.' He did find it, in Norway. No one who does not have the alphabet at his command or hidden away somewhere in the recesses of his brain can possibly do this. The deadlock had gone.

Third, the patient will probably not be able to learn as a child learns. The teacher's job is somehow to find the key to unlock the knowledge that he already has, to bring it out of the darkness.

For instance, it will probably be no good to say, Today we will learn the word "carpet".' But if instead you discuss together, at length and over several lessons, all that you know or can find out about carpets, then slowly the word has a chance of seeping into his 'instinctive' vocabulary. A carpet is warming, deadens noise, is colourful and cosy. They are made all over the world. Wonderful ones are handmade in Persia. There are magic carpets and praying carpets, fitted, rich and worn ones. Arabs spread them on the desert sand, we lay them on our floors. All spell a little luxury, a little of civilization's softening up process. One can speak of a carpet of flowers; Raleigh laid his cloak as a carpet for Queen Elizabeth; a bride steps on a ceremonial strip of carpet as she emerges from church. And so on, using every scrap of imagination and ingenuity that you can summon up.

Lastly, and much the most vital, the patient is bored, bored to tears, bored to death. So the teacher has to base his whole method on alleviating this most numbing of all human conditions. Try to get him interested in anything from gardening to pets, from painting to music. Explore with him his hobbies, be they baseball or philately, carpentry or numismatics. You will know many things that help, but perhaps occupation, purpose and a little happiness are good antidotes to boredom.

It is good to have these antidotes uppermost in your mind when you start your first lesson.

A Stroke in the Family

Planning the first lesson

So you might begin with a few games, getting as much communication as is possible between patient and teacher as you play, and also finding out a good deal about how much the patient can manage.

Recognising colours and shapes

Dominoes, if he has played it before, may be the easiest. Straightaway you will see whether he can recognize and put two identical numbers together, like this:

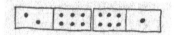

This doesn't tell you if he could do it with the word 'six' or the figure '6', but nevertheless you have learnt something. In ludo he has to be able to count the numbers on each dice, add them together, then move his counter along the board an equivalent amount. This is one stage further in his understanding of figures.

In order to play checkers (draughts) he must form a plan, try to outwit his opponent, and notice when he is in a position to whip some counters from the enemy ranks.

In the early stages of teaching, Pat fell for dominoes and Alan for ludo. Both managed well and they found they were on equal footing with their opponents. It was their first effort at solving a simple problem.

Jigsaw puzzles and simple card games are first rate occupations. Amongst many good things, they have the merit that the patient can try them later on his own, and help prevent his sitting staring into space.

The identification of shapes is connected to intelligence and with these two games you will discover how much the patient can manage.

I tried, first, cutting up a magazine picture into about ten pieces. Both Pat and Alan put it together well. Then we bought some small jigsaws, not those for children, but 30 or 40 piece jigsaws for adults, with a clear picture. Later, as soon as one of these was done without help, we bought one with 50-60 pieces, and so on - increasing the size and difficulty all the time.

Card games (patience or a game for two people) pose a more difficult problem. Can the patient identify red from black? Can he work out the value of the cards? Can he tell the shape of a club ♣ from a spade ♠ or a heart ♡ from a diamond ◇ ?

To give you some idea of the progress that Pat and Alan achieved let me tell you this: At the beginning both of them were only able to note the difference between black and red, court card from number card, nothing else. Now they both play very reasonable bridge.

At this time you could put in front of the patient a box of chalks or anything that shows all the colours. Ask him to pick up the yellow one, the blue, etc.

Memory and observation
Since memory and observation are also problems we found it worth while to put some items on a tray covered with a cloth; say a pen, a cup, a box of matches, a book and a key. Show them to him, then cover the tray and get him to communicate to you (via speech, writing, drawing or gestures, whatever he can manage) what is on the

tray. Gradually you can increase the number of things on the tray and lessen the length of time he is allowed to look at it.

You can try a little mental arithmetic:

$4 + 8 = ?$	$37 - 6 = ?$
$21 + 7 = ?$	$7 + 4 + 3 = ?$
$18 - 9 = ?$	$8 \times 2 = ?$

Again he must solve the problem and communicate the answer to you.

It was fun for us to note that whilst Alan could knock Pat into a cocked hat over the jigsaws, Pat had a most surprising flair for mental arithmetic.

It is worth while to concentrate on getting the patient to both observe and picture things.

Pat's ability to observe was poor. She looked but she did not see. So, amongst many things, I sketched out an empty map of our village and Pat had to plod up and down the High Street writing in (or communicating so that others could write in) all that she saw. It took her many hours, but she made it.

Alan - the brilliant author - had trained all his powers to note things in words and, as a result, his picturing of things was poor. Yet to memorize words without pictures is difficult for all of us, let alone for the stroke patient. So I would build up a little word picture, something like this: 'In the foreground is a lovely garden with roses, a pool and a lawn. Large trees frame the garden and are outlined against the blue sky. Swallows fly past and blackbirds peck for worms in the grass.' Or: 'The streets are far below us as we look out of the window. It is a toy town. Cars would fit into match boxes, and half-a-dozen people could stand in the palm of my hand. Children scurry like money spiders behind their parents.' Then I would get Alan to shut his eyes, picture it, and draw the result.

In doing these things, and anything else you can think of on these lines, you have already begun to tackle many subjects: getting through to the patient; making him concentrate; gaining his interest; getting him observing, thinking, picturing, solving problems; helping him to identify shapes, numbers and colours.

And most important of all, perhaps you are on your way to a mutual understanding.

Example lessons

Here are two examples of complete lessons which we gave at this stage. All lessons must be fully prepared beforehand.

In almost all cases I have given two examples of lessons at the end of each chapter and two further examples, of the same standard, in the appendixes. These examples give you a sample of everything I found most fruitful with Pat and Alan.

Lesson 1
(1) Go through the general idea that is involved with each of these games and their equipment: dominoes, ludo, checkers (draughts) and playing cards.

DOMINOES
(a) Look at the dominoes and mark the different number of dots on each half.
(b) Match up the numbers and discuss the procedure.

LUDO

(a) Look at the dice and mark the number of dots on each side. Try throwing a pair.

(b) Check the aim and object of the game.

(c) Move the counters in accordance with the total of the two dice thrown.

CHECKERS

(a) Note the two coloured counters and alternate black and white squares of the board.

(b) Discuss how it is played.

PLAYING CARDS

(a) Sort out the 52 cards into suits and seniority.

(b) Discuss the shapes, colours, court cards, aces and number cards.

(2) Hand over an already cut up magazine picture and get the patient to put it together as if it were a jigsaw.

(3) Using a box of coloured chalks, ask the patient to pick up the red, green, yellow, etc.

(4) Uncover the tray on which are a pencil, a knife and a book. Get him to study it, then recover the tray and see whether he remembers the objects and can communicate to you what they were.

(5) Ask what is missing in these three sketches:

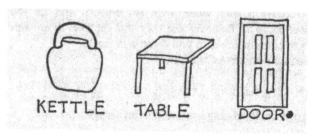

KETTLE   TABLE   DOOR

(6) Read out the following and get the patient to draw a picture of it afterwards:

'A child was playing on the beach. He had built a sand castle and put an upturned bucket on the top. Around the castle was a moat which he was busy trying to fill with sea water.'

(7) Play a game of dominoes, ludo or checkers, whichever the patient seemed most at home with at the start of the lesson.

HOMEWORK

Leave magazine picture jigsaws for him to assemble.

Lesson 2

(1) Sort out a number of playing cards into suits and seniority.

(2) Call out Ace of spades, 4 of diamonds, 8 of spades Jack of hearts, 9 of hearts, 2 of clubs, for the patient to pick out of the spread pack.

(3) Play a short game of patience together.

(4) Do a magazine picture jigsaw, this time cut into smaller pieces and more awkward shapes.

(5) Uncover a tray laden with six objects, and let the patient study it. Recover the tray and get him to remember and communicate to you what was there.

(6) Mental arithmetic. Ask him:

4 + 2	12 - 2	2 x 10
7 + 11	4 + 4 + 1	31 + 9

(7) Ask what is missing in the following three lines:

   (a) 2. 4. 6. 10. 12.

   (b) D. E. F. H. I.

   (c) ◇ ♡ ♤

(8) Work with colours. Give him the crayons.

    (a) What colour is grass?

    (b) What colour is the sky?

    (c) What colour is a flame?

    (d) Red and yellow = ?

    (e) Blue and yellow = ?

    (f) Red and blue = ?

(9) Play dominoes, ludo or checkers, preferably a different one from the last lesson but the choice dependent on progress and wish.

HOMEWORK

A 30 piece jigsaw. Two more sample lessons are given in Appendix 1

4 - Discovering where to start

The major problem to be dealt with is words - the spoken, heard, read and written word through which we communicate and understand. By playing the games you will have begun to discover some of the patient's limitations. Now you must probe further and start helping at the bottom rung of the ladder of words.

Does he understand as you talk slowly and carefully to him?

Can he follow the meaning when several people are talking to each other?

Does he understand if you read to him?

Can he read on his own?

Can he read aloud?

Can he talk at all? Has he a total vocabulary of four words? More?

Has he an apparently 'instinctive' small vocabulary but no ability to say any one particular word he wants to say? For instance, can he manage with no trouble at all this conversation: 'How are you?' 'I'm very well, thank you. And you?" 'Fine, thanks. Isn't it a lovely day?' 'Marvellous. Really marvellous.' Yet should you ask him to say the words 'very well' or 'really marvellous' in an unfamiliar context, he cannot.

Does he mix up words or invent his own?

Can he write on his own? A letter? A word? A sentence?

Does he find a word like 'afforestation' easy and an abstract word like 'from' impossible?

A Stroke in the Family

Can he copy out the written word (left handed if necessary)?

The rung of the ladder was different for Pat and Alan, but with both the fight to re-familiarize themselves with words had to start at an acutely simple level.

'Re-familiarize' is a clumsy verb, yet it is important to realize that this is the basis of what you are trying to do. Neither Pat nor Alan could learn as a child learns, but they could dig their own hidden knowledge out into the daylight.

Blue Peter time

It is worth hunting up some well written sentences where both the words and the meanings are clear and simple. Get the patient to try reading it on his own, then read it to him, and finally read it aloud together. He can then try his hand at communicating to you the meaning of the sentence. Push, push for this effort at communication. Get him to try words, gestures, drawings, pointing at things, miming. (Pat, of course, found the acting right up her street.) But even if he cannot act don't let him give up. It's your will against his. He must and he will tell you. A stroke does not damage a sense of humour, so this can lead to laughter. I wish you could have seen Alan Moorehead, the author, competing for Pat's Oscar!

You can also try having two copies of some short page. As you read aloud from your copy the patient follows on his.

On twenty four separate pieces of paper draw a dozen objects and their names, like this:

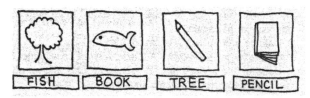

Then get the patient to match name to object. Alternatively, tear out some magazine pictures, write out a heading for each one or a brief descriptive sentence, and get him to match words to pictures.

Write out a few letters and ask him to find as many words as possible using only these letters. For example:

FTRO		HETCA		
To	Tor	Cat	The	Heat
Of	Rot	He	Tea	Hate
For	Fort	Het	Ace	Teach
Or		At	Hat	

For another version of this, now with the meaning attached, give him an anagram as you find them in crossword puzzles. For example:

An animal (anagram of TCA)

Something that grows in the earth (anagram of RETE)

Then move on to more difficult ones as the patient progresses.

Write out a sentence on a strip of paper, making capitals and punctuation clear. Cut it up so that each word is on a separate piece. Then get the patient to put the sentence in order. 'The house is by the sea.' You may find, as we did, that you'll need hundreds of these.

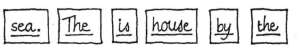

Eventually you will be able to mix two sentences together for him to assemble correctly.

For instance:

'The weather is hot and dry. The garden needs watering'.

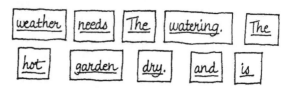

Think of a word, say 'table', and see if the patient can find it in the dictionary. To begin with we found it helpful to print the word clearly so that he can keep referring to it, letter by letter, as he hunts. When he has found it, read out the meaning together.

Similarly, you can hand him a closed atlas and ask him to point to Moscow, New York, etc. If he fails to find it, get him to look it up in the index at the back. When he has found the word, get him to read the reference, page 24 D.C., then turn to page 24 and hunt for it in the square marked D.C.

At any time in the first half of the lesson write out a word, a few words or a sentence and get the patient to study it and picture the meaning, then put it to one side. At the end of the lesson see if he can remember and speak or draw what it was.

Sometimes it is helpful to ally words to actions as well as to pictures. This, done perhaps in the middle of a lesson, makes a welcome relief from sitting at a table. Get the patient to copy both your actions and the words you say to describe them. 'I stand up.' 'We walk.' 'We walk up and down the room.' 'You sit.' 'Hand me the black pencil.' And so on. Do the actions and say the words in unison. Two people bobbing about the room has an element of slapstick about it. It's funny, relaxing, with a built-in value of its own.

Sitting down again at the table, pick up a couple of objects, say a book and a pen, and have your first crack at the little words. 'The pen is ON the book.' 'The pen is BY the book.' 'The book is UNDER the pen.' 'I'm holding the pen ABOVE the book.' And so on. Do the actions as you speak the words.

Alan, particularly, liked to have as many drawings as could be managed, with the names of the object or the action printed clearly by the side. If drawing is a closed book to you, find uncluttered pictures and print on them. But I think you will find your own efforts at sketching, however amateur, will interest and amuse him more than a 'set piece'. Also in your own sketch you can choose the words you want stressed. Here are a few examples:

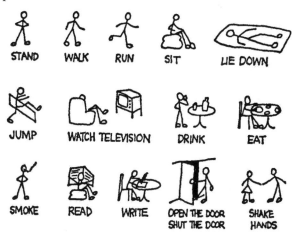

STAND   WALK   RUN   SIT   LIE DOWN

JUMP   WATCH TELEVISION   DRINK   EAT

SMOKE   READ   WRITE   OPEN THE DOOR SHUT THE DOOR   SHAKE HANDS

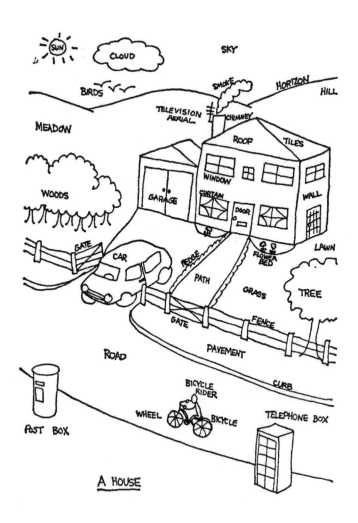

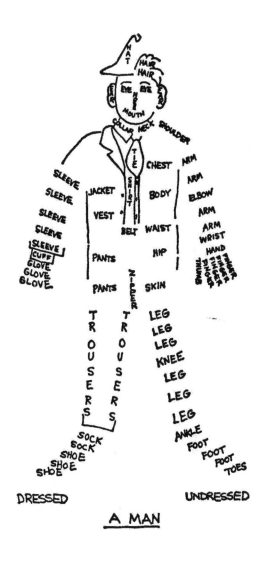

A MAN

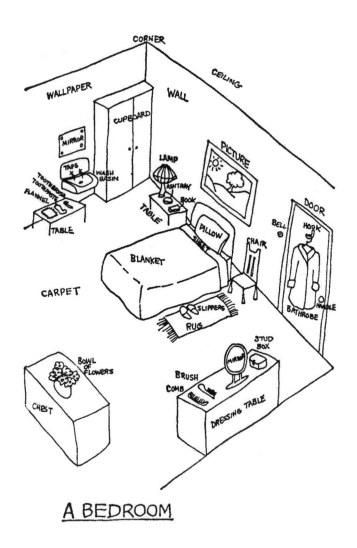

A BEDROOM

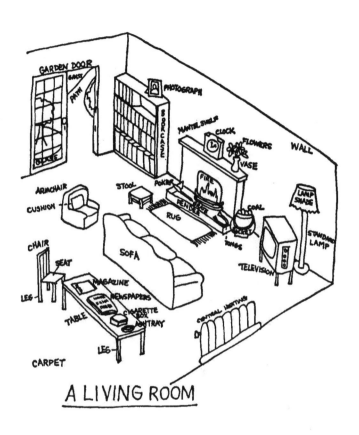

A LIVING ROOM

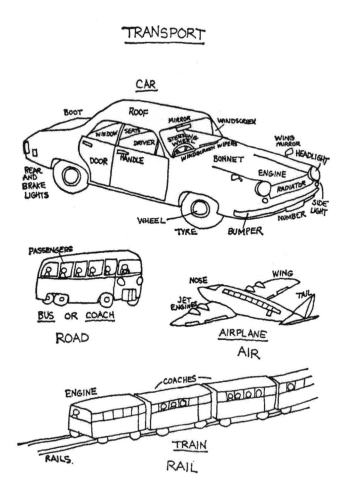

TRANSPORT

CAR

BUS OR COACH

ROAD

AIRPLANE

AIR

TRAIN

RAIL

4 - Discovering where to start

The work in this chapter is all fairly simple. And some of the things can be done when the patient is on his own, as homework. Jigsaws come in useful here as well, and the television. Leaving him something to do is, I think, of value. It cannot be stressed too often how destroying it is to a stroke patient to be left twiddling his thumbs.

Also at this and every stage Roald Dahl and Lucy Moorehead found the importance of taking Pat and Alan around and about, ensuring that stimulus in one form or another was always present.

One must, of course, study the need of each individual. In Alan's case Lucy had to protect him a little from overwork once the teaching had begun. All his life he had been a tremendous worker. He tended to tire himself by doing the homework for too long periods. But Alan will probably be a great exception. It is rare to find anyone so used to long periods of determined concentration. It was different with Pat. She is an actress. Actresses work only when they are given lines. Inertia and apathy were deadweight burdens and Roald had to jog us to keep her busy, busy, busy.

Before going on to the next stage, it must be mentioned here that, for all the teaching, it is still the husband, wife (relation or friend, whoever is in command), it is still this one person who can make or break. This is the most difficult job in the world, for he has to act as shield, morale booster, guide and egger-on in the 'cruel-to-be-kind' fashion. And he has to have courage, understanding, sympathy, patience, and an instinct for when to push and when to let up. The load on him is heavy. But a team of good teachers will relieve it enormously.

A Stroke in the Family

Here are two examples of complete lessons which we gave at this stage:

Lesson 1

(1) Read aloud, then together, the following paragraph:
'It was six o'clock on a summer's evening. There were long shadows on the grass and the air was filled with the scent of roses.'

Then put it to one side and ask the patient to communicate to you the meaning.

2) Fit the pictures and words to one another.

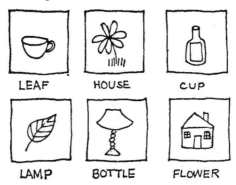

(3) Make as many words as possible from these letters:
AIPNL.

(4) Find an anagram of RDEAB that means something to eat.

(5) Make sentences out of the following groups of words:

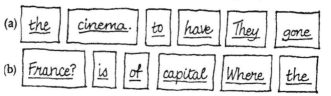

6) Find the following words in the dictionary:
Good

Tennis

Street

Car

Then read out the meaning together.

HOMEWORK

(1)   Study this drawing with the words printed on it. (Drawing given to the patient.)

(2)   Find as many words as possible from ESHDA and from PRTAE.

Lesson 2

(1) Study and try to learn the following:

'Lunch is ready.'

(2) Take a match and a match-box. Do the actions (and get the patient to do them) as you say the following sentences:

The match is IN the box.

The match is UNDER the box.

The match is ON the box.

The match is NEAR the box.

The match is taken OUT of the box.

The match is taken TO the box.

The match is taken FROM the box.

The match is moved OVER the box.

(3) Using an atlas, ask the patient to point to:

Paris   What country is it in?

Rome   How old is this city?

New York Is it the capital of the U.S.A.?

Mexico   Do they speak Italian here?

The Nile Is it a useful river? Why?

Edinburgh What is the national dress of the Scots?

and ask the questions after each place has been found. Look up anything unknown and trace its whereabouts from the reference given in the index.

(4) Get up and do the appropriate actions together as you say the following words:

We get up.
I sit down.
We walk about the room.
You open the window.
I shut the door.
I fall over.
You move the chair.

(5) Arrange these words so that they make sense:

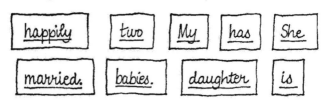

(6) See if the patient can remember the words he studied at the start of the lesson ('Lunch is ready').

HOMEWORK

(1) Give him six groups of words to make into six sentences.

(2) Find the correct sentence by unmixing these words:
EW RAE OIGNG OT A MLIF.

Two more sample lessons are given in Appendix 2.

5 - Maintaining the patient's interest

After several weeks of teaching any reserve that existed between patient and teacher should be well on the way out. It is important to work for this, as any feelings of shame, inferiority or fear of facing the facts on the part of the patient will hinder and worry him. It is not his fault or his weakness. It might have been you or me.

You will find constant repetition is essential. To achieve this a little cunning is needed, for the repetition must not lead to boredom. Snap from one subject to another, twisting everything round to give variation. Use most often the exercises that combine profit and fun.

Let the patient correct your errors

The patient's lack of confidence must be your concern. A few little triumphs work magic. For instance, I asked Pat one day, 'Where is Washington?' She pointed to the northwest coast of the United States, and I shook my head. Whereupon, with great gusto, she explained the difference between Washington State and Washington D.C. One up for her. On another occasion I asked Alan, 'Where was Christopher Colombus born? He answered, 'Genoa,' and again I shook my head, thinking that it was somewhere at least in the Iberian peninsula. We hunted it up in an encyclopedia, and of course he was right. Alan also regularly corrects my atrocious spelling. A triumph each time. Teachers who are first class spellers should make a few mistakes on purpose. And indeed I found it very helpful to set exercises where the patient had to correct mistakes in sentences

A Stroke in the Family

For example:

(1) There are 48 hours in a day.

(2) Mary and John is very happy.

(3) David has written seven book.

(4) Anne likes cooking but he hates washing up.

(5) Oslo is the capital of Sweden.

(6) The pencil has run out of ink.

As both you and the patient progress a little with your joint task, it is worth while trying more difficult material. You must always move forward, only leaving to later anything that is impossible at the moment.

Widen the search for the patient's interests

Are you sure you know all his interests? It is important because, using these interests, you can steer a harder course with greater ease and enjoyment.

One way of discovering this is to use reference books. Had you looked in at many of the sessions with Pat or Alan you might have thought we intended writing a learned history of the world, so loaded was our table with massive volumes of knowledge!

Try turning over the pages of an encyclopedia, and stopping at any item that catches the attention of the patient. Read it out to him and read it aloud with him. Let him read it alone, if this is possible. Ask him questions about it, to be answered (and they must be answered) with speech, writing, gestures, however he can best communicate. Look up in a dictionary the meaning of some of the words that he is interested in. And again read it aloud with him.

If you find he has a passion for football, lawn tennis,

chess, the works of a painter, any famous man, or what-ever, try to get a book or pamphlet that concerns this subject.

The patient may be interested in daily affairs. And in this connection he may be worried that he is getting 'out of the swim'. In which case have a newspaper handy and help him to read and understand what is taking place. He may like the comics or cartoons. Fine. Go through them with him. The sports results may be important to him, the stock market, the gossip column, the critics. Try them all and work through them with him.

Change location or 'props'

Another idea for a change in the middle of a lesson is to get up and wander round the house. You can talk as you go, about the things you see. Something needs painting, a plant is just coming into bloom, a migrant bird has arrived, anything, everything. And encourage him to observe for himself and point out things to you.

When you return to your workroom you might get out a typewriter. Can the patient pick out the letters? Can he type his own name? Can he copy a sentence? If a hand is handicapped, a typewriter is a useful possession. It needs only one finger of his good hand! But should a hand be only partially afflicted, then using it will do him good.

To assist his memory we found it helpful to revert to the object laden tray again. Only this time, as well as several objects, you write out their names on separate pieces of paper and put these, too, on the tray. Give him a moment, or longer, to study it. Then see whether he can remember the objects and words, and match them up.

You can work out a very simple crossword for the patient to do, first during the lesson and later on his own. If you put in a one word clue, say the word FALSE, he can look it up in the dictionary. There he will see the word WRONG, and this is the answer. It is perhaps beneficial to give all types of clues, not only the word to look up in the dictionary but also anagrams, words he has a chance of knowing, sentences where the word omitted is the answer, geographical names where he can use an atlas if necessary to find the answer. You can choose the clues and the answers according to the patient's capabilities and also according to the words you have recently been working with.

We have composed hundreds of these, of all standards and sizes, and we find it easiest to start with a set pattern of black and white squares, perhaps like this:

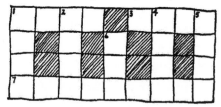

Or, later, like this:

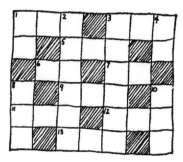

5 - Maintaining the patient's interest

Below is an early example. As you will see, a few letters are already printed in, then omitted as he grows used to trying crosswords and gets better at doing them.

(For Pat)

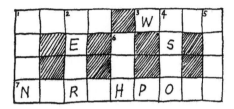

	Across		Down
1	Your surname	1	'Jack fell ---- and broke his crown.'
3	A wild animal that is like a dog and hunts in packs	2	To perceive by ear. (An anagram of R H A E.)
7	(2 words of 5 and 4 letters each) The extreme top of the world	4	The capital of Norway.
		5	A number.
		6	A tree. Also the burnt out embers of a fire or cigarette.

(*Note by Roald Dahl: For at least a year, Val made one crossword a day for Pat to do.*)

Overleaf is an example of a more difficult crossword, intentionally worked out so that there are plenty of small words. It is also of value to make up a larger type of crossword that mainly comprises the particular subject you are working on at the time.

Here are two completed examples (clues should still be clear and simple).

A Stroke in the Family

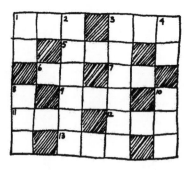

Across

1 You can go in and --- of a door

3 A Number

5 His Royal Highness (initials)

6 It is either right -- wrong

7 Peas grow -- a pod

9 You hear with this, one being on the left of your head and the other on he right

11 A drink (anagram of L E A)

12 Another drink, made from leaves

13 Timid (anagram of H Y S)

Down

1 The stamp is stuck -- the envelope

2 Ones, twos, ------, fours

3 8 + 9 + 15 - 2

4 He won by the skin - - his teeth

8 Vermin, like a large mouse

10 He was a --- man, weighing 200 lbs. (Anagram of T F A)

(1) Colour and Light

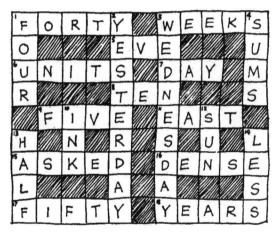

(2) Numbers and Time

To begin with, crosswords such as these last two are probably better attempted during a lesson. Later, as the patient advances, they do well as homework.

Overleaf is an example of a lesson we gave when working on these ideas:

A Stroke in the Family

Lesson 1

(1) Get out a typewriter. See whether the patient can copy out a word or type his own name from memory. Dictate some words and see whether he can type them.

(2) Get him to type a sentence, copied from a book, or one you have made up. Say, 'The time is four o'clock,' Then get him to study it and try to learn it.

(3) Do this crossword (made for Alan) together:

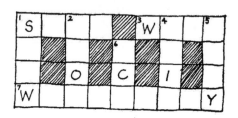

Across

1 Out of danger. an anagram of F S E A
3 'How are you?' 'I am very ----, thank you'
7 A day of the week

Down

1 This can fall from the sky in winter, and people ski on it
2 You eat this
4 A girl's name
5 Your wife's name, an anagram of D N E L
6 Number One in a pack of cards

(4) Uncover a tray on which are six objects and six slips of paper with the name of each of the objects written out separately. Get him to match name to object, then remember both after the tray is hidden.

(5) Look through one item in a newspaper.

(6) Ask him to correct the error in these sentences:

    (a) He smokes ten cigarettes a day.

    (b) There are 31 days in every month.

    (c) A brightly burning fire is cold.

    (d) How are you

    (e) Every man has two foot.

    (f) They has four children.

(7) See whether he still remembers the sentence he typed.

('The time is four o'clock.')

HOMEWORK

Crossword.

Two more sample lessons are given in Appendix 3.

6 - Depression and loss of confidence

Up to this time we found we had worked with words a great deal, but had not pressed the patient to find his own words unaided.

Before going on to discuss further steps in therapy, I would like to take a longer look into the problems of depression and self confidence. These problems are yours as well as his. For make no mistake about it, this is something you are going to have to cope with. You are going to have to be strong, patient and understanding. A lack of consideration for others can be one of the results of despair.

Depression

If you put yourself in the patient's place, you will see that he is bound to have black moods of depression.

We feel that to deny him, as it were, the right to despondency is a mistake. If anyone ever had cause to feel depressed it is the victim of a bad stroke. So perhaps it is best to go gently about helping him dispel these moods when they occur. Provide some of his 'favourites', saved for a rainy day. Simple things are fine. Play his favourite game or record, give him his favourite food, talk to him about the things or people he likes, don't leave him alone, ask in a good friend, take him to a film. This is neither to pander to his misery nor to order cheerfulness too briskly. If he can manage to talk or communicate in any way and he wants to discuss his troubles, good. Let him talk about anything, however drastic, strange or dangerous seeming the subject may be. As with you or me the old cliche may work - to share is to halve. Besides, in this mood, his very need will force him to try to communicate, and this is just what is wanted.

Loss of Confidence

Lack of confidence is a less spectacular but more permanent condition and it is vital to try to help it. The biggest answer to it that we have discovered is to keep the person occupied. Encourage him to do every single thing he is able to do for himself. Clean shoes, stir the soup, post letters. And, of course, work at his lessons. With any luck the little round-about-the-house jobs will help keep at bay the deadly feeling of uselessness; and there is nothing like being able to work hard for your own recovery. There are small things like always bringing him into a conversation or decision, not talking about him to others as if he were not there, giving him loads of time to get what he wants to say across; but you will know of these. And you could try leaving him on his own with a child. (*Note by Roald Dahl: This is terrific.*) Children have a means of communication that is all their own and in our opinion they can possess a magic touch with a stroke patient. The very qualities of childhood that are lost at puberty meet him halfway. It is by no means child to child; but it is something like soul to soul. With both Pat and Alan we would get a child of, say, five or eight to come in during a lesson. Then, on some pretext, the teacher would go out of the room. Five seconds later patient and child could be heard talking away together, engrossed, uninhibited, and at ease with each other.

6 - Depression and loss of confidence

Finding his own words

To return, now, to the lessons that involve helping the patient to find his own words. You will soon discover, or probably know already, whether these words will come easier spoken or written. Both of course are important, but the spoken word must have priority. We tried many different ways of getting at this. You can write out a list of sentences, leaving out the word you want the patient to supply. For example:

(1) He is reading a - - - -
(2) The sky is - - - - our heads.
(3) The man is - - - - - - - a letter with a pen.
(4) The phone is - - - - - - -
(5) He - - - - - - cigars
(6) I would like a - - - - - of water.

Ask him for a word that has the opposite meaning to 'old', 'fat', 'dark', 'happy', etc.

Get him to think of something, anything, that is black, heavy, good to eat, green, wet; something that can be sharpened, washed, listened to, watched, and so on.

Give him two or three words, say, 'phone' and 'ring', or 'paper', 'read' and 'glasses', and see whether he can make up a sentence using these words.

Ask him to think of another word meaning the same as 'pale', 'hard', 'deep blue', etc.

See if he can find any suitable word to describe a man, a house, a garden. For instance, he could say 'a tall man', 'a big house', 'a lovely garden'.

May we give you a word of warning here, as we learned it from Pat and Alan. It is best not to mention grammar, nor even to think of words in this sense. In other words, do not ask him to find an adjective that can suitably be put before the noun 'man', but ask him to find a word that describes 'man'. It is a small but important difference. Give him a list of words like 'bell', 'walk', 'fight', and see if he can produce words that rhyme with them.

Can he reproduce animal sounds or sounds of any sort? Ask him what noise a sheep makes, or a bell or a bird.

Ask him short questions. 'Where does wool come from?' 'What did you have for supper last night?'

Read sentences with him that you have already written out, the complete sentence this time. Repeat this several times, then suddenly fade out your own voice. You may find he will complete it on his own.

Try a short piece of dictation, a word, a phrase, a sentence, to see whether he can write it down. Give him plenty of time and repeat it many times. You may find he suddenly says the words, almost without knowing he is doing it! I think the reason for this is that his whole mind is struggling to write the word, so he is freed from any stress as to how to say it - and out come the words.

Taped lessons

At about this stage of work we started using a tape recorder as a means of doing work at home when the teacher is gone, gradually building up a little 'library' of lessons available to him at any time. We found it essential to have the lessons written out for him, as well as spoken on the tape, as they do in the Linguaphone series.

It is not easy to work from so impersonal a source,

indeed Alan found it very difficult, but nevertheless the tape recorder has many values, perhaps the most important one being that the patient can wind back the tape at will to get a repetition of any part he finds hard.

The following is an example of a recording I made. All four lessons fitted on to one twenty-minute tape. Note the constant repetition which is essential:

Tape 1. Lesson 1
Will you say the first sentence with me? Ready?
(1) The car is outside the door.

Again. 'The car is outside the door.' And again. 'The car is outside the door.' Now will you say it once more with me, then say it aloud by yourself? Ready? 'The car is outside the door.' (Long pause.) Will you say the second sentence with me? Ready?
(2) I will answer the phone.

Again. 'I will answer the phone.' And again. 'I will answer the phone.' Now will you say it once more with me, then say it aloud by yourself? Ready? 'I will answer the phone.' (Long pause.) Will you read the third sentence with me? Ready?
(3) The T.V. was bad last night.

Again. The T.V. was bad last night.' And again. 'The T.V. was bad last night.' Now will you say it once more with me, then say it aloud by yourself? Ready? 'The T.V. was bad last night.' (Long pause.) Will you read the fourth sentence with me? Ready?
(4) The small boy reads well.

Again. 'The small boy reads well.' And again. 'The small boy reads well.' Now will you say it once more with me, then say it aloud by yourself? Ready? 'The small boy reads well.' (Long pause.) Will you read the fifth sentence with me? Ready?

(5) You must write him a letter.

Again. 'You must write him a letter.' And again. 'You must write him a letter.' Now will you say it once more with me, then say it aloud by yourself? Ready? 'You must write him a letter.' (Long pause.)

Will you read the sixth sentence with me? Ready?

(6) It is cold and wet outside.

Again. 'It is cold and wet outside.' And again. 'It is cold and wet outside.' Now will you say it once more with me, then say it aloud by yourself? Ready? 'It is cold and wet outside.' (Long pause.) Will you read the seventh sentence with me? Ready?

(7) The room is too hot.

Again. 'The room is too hot.' And again. 'The room is too hot.' Now will you say it once more with me, then say it aloud by yourself? Ready? 'The room is too hot.' (Long pause.) Will you read the eighth sentence with me? Ready?

(8) I have a good book to read.

Again. 'I have a good book to read.' And again. 'I have a good book to read.' Now will you say it once more with me, then say it aloud by yourself? Ready? 'I have a good book to read.' (Long pause.)

Now let's read all these eight sentences through together, one after the other. Ready?

(1) The car is outside the door.

(2) I will answer the phone.

(3) The T.V. was bad last night.

(4) The small boy reads well.

(5) You must write him a letter.

(6) It is cold and wet outside.

(7) The room is too hot.

(8) I have a good book to read.

Tape 1 Lesson 2

This is a sound you find difficult to say. The letters that make the sound are S followed by H. SH. SH. If you remember, we found that you could say this sound well if you think of it in terms of shutting someone up. Imagine you are talking on the telephone and someone in the room is talking. You turn to them and say, 'Sh! Sh!'

Let's try it. Ready? 'Sh.' Again. 'Sh.' And again. 'Sh.'

Now let's say the words on your list. Ready? 'Sheep.' Again. 'Sheep.' And again. 'Sheep.' Now try it once more with me, then say it aloud by yourself. Ready? 'Sheep.' (Pause.)

Now let's say the second,word. Ready? 'Shoe.' Again. 'Shoe.' And again. 'Shoe.' Now try it once more with me, then say it aloud by yourself. Ready? 'Shoe.' (Pause.)

Now let's say the third word. Ready? 'Fish.' Again. 'Fish.' And again. 'Fish.' Now let's try it once more with me, then you say it aloud by yourself. Ready? 'Fish.' (Pause.)

Now let's say the last word. Ready? 'Dash.' Again. 'Dash.' And again. 'Dash.' Now try it once more with me, then you say it aloud by yourself. Ready? 'Dash.' (Pause.)

A Stroke in the Family

Tape 1 Lesson 3

In the following six sentences there is a word left out from each. Will you say the first sentence with me, and try to put in the missing word? Ready?

(1) The match is - the box.

Again. The match is - the box.' And again. 'The match is - the box.' Now will you look up the written answer and we will say the complete sentence through together again? Ready? 'The match is in the box.' Now the second sentence. Ready?

(2) The paper is - the desk.

Again. 'The paper is - the desk.' And again. 'The paper is - the desk.' Now will you look up the written answer and we will say the complete sentence through together again? Ready? 'The paper is on the desk.' Now the third sentence. Ready?

(3) The dog jumped - the fence.

Again. 'The dog jumped - the fence.' And again. 'The dog jumped - the fence.' Now will you look up the written answer and we will say the complete sentence through together again? Ready? 'The dog jumped over the fence.' Now the fourth sentence. Ready?

(4) The cat sat - the fire.

Again. 'The cat sat - the fire.' And again. 'The cat sat - the fire.' Now will you look up the written answer and we will say the complete sentence through together again? Ready? 'The cat sat by the fire.' Now the fifth sentence. Ready?

(5) The grass grows - the tree.

Again. 'The grass grows - the tree.' And again. The grass grows - the tree.' Now will you look up the written answer and we will say the complete sentence through together again? Ready? 'The grass grows under the tree.' Now the sixth and last sentence. Ready?

(6) The ball went - the hoop.

Again. The ball went - the hoop.' And again. The ball went - the hoop.' Now will you look up the written answer and we will say the complete sentence through together again? Ready? The ball went through the hoop.'

Tape 1 Lesson 4

Will you read with me the paragraph in front of you? First slowly, then a second time a little quicker. Ready?

'It was extraordinary weather. The rainbird, a small lilac breasted cuckoo, followed us everywhere. I never did succeed in catching sight of the bird itself, but we woke each morning to the sound of its mournful three note cry. It went on and on, and it was never wrong. By midday black clouds had piled up over the sun, and in the evening a thunderstorm would burst on top of us. Where normally in January or February we should have been covered in dust, we travelled now in deep black mud with chains on the wheels, and sometimes three hours would go by while we cut down trees and made causeways across the rivers.' (From *No Room in the Ark* by Alan Moorehead)

During these lessons the patient had the following written out in front of him:

Lesson 1

(1) The car is outside the door.

(2) I will answer the phone.

(3) The T.V. was bad last night

(4) The small boy reads well.

(5) You must write him a letter.

(6) It is cold and wet outside.

(7) The room is too hot.

(8) I have a good book to read.

Lesson 2

SH.   Sh!   Sh!

Sheep Shoe

Fish Dash

Lesson 3

(These strips of paper were cut and folded for the patient to refer to)

(1) The match is - the box.

(2) The paper is - the desk.

(3) The dog jumped - the fence.

(4) The cat sat - the fire.

(5) The grass grows - the tree.

(6) The ball went - the hoop.

Lesson 4

For Lesson 4, he had an extract from *No Room in the Ark*.

6 - Depression and loss of confidence

Here I must mention the problem of getting the patient to do homework.

Some Homework

Every stroke patient needs a different approach, different lessons, different treatment. And he will surely react in his own way to the idea of working on his own. As far as we were concerned, Pat and Alan were at the opposite ends of the pole. No one could stop Alan working, and a team of wild horses was needed to spark Pat into making an effort.

Alan's case - almost certainly the rarer of the two extremes - was easier to manage.

Pat was a problem. However much she really intended getting down to the homework, when the time came the inertia beat down her will power. As with so many things, we did not solve this problem. But we did learn some dodges that helped a little.

Roald made a habit of breezing frequently through the room where Pat was working. As he passed her he would stop, look at the progress, and encourage.

We soon learnt which exercises Pat preferred to do, and we concentrated on these. As soon as she arrived for the next lesson we asked to see the homework. Pat, honest as the day is long, would tell or show us what little she had managed. Contrition would show on her face, for Pat likes to please. And this acted as the smallest of spurs.

Also - a thoroughly dirty trick, this - I would phone her at the times when I'd learned her apathy would be at its worst. How was the homework going? What had she done? Just sometimes the keenness of someone else would goad her onward.

These are only small contributions, but they were of help. You will think of others that suit your individual case.

Here are two examples of lessons we gave at this stage:

Lesson 1

(1) Fill in the missing words:

    (a) A seesaw goes - and - .

    (b) It is too hot. Please - the window.

    (c) The car is travelling at 70 miles per - .

    (d) You get tanned if you bathe.

    (e) My sight is poor so I wear - .

    (f) We use a - and fork to eat with.

(2) Find a word you can associate with each of the following:

Cat	Food	Flower
Sun	Grey	Hand
Green	Light	Fire
Book	Water	Wine

(3) Read these sentences together several times, then fade out your voice:

    (1) The phone is ringing.

    (2) I want to read the papers.

    (3) Where is my book?

    (4) The meal is ready.

    (5) Will you have a cigarette?

    (6) It is fine today.

Then get the patient to try and memorize the last sentence.

6 - Depression and loss of confidence

(4) Read together and discuss a selected short column from a daily newspaper.

(5) Quickly answer yes or no to these questions:

    (1) Is Mary a boy's name?

    (2) Is it cold today?

    (3) Did you go out last night?

    (4) Does 2 + 3 + 4 = 9?

    (5) Is Wednesday the second day of the week?

    (6) Was Goya a painter?

(6) Write each word of this sentence on a separate bit of paper:

    'John and Jenny will marry in March'.

Take the paper with 'Jenny' on it out and hand the rest to the patient to assemble in order. Tell him of the missing word, and see whether he can add a suitable one for himself to complete the sentence.

(7) Find out whether he has been able to memorize the sentence learned earlier. ('It is fine today.')

HOMEWORK

    Lessons 1 and 2 on the tape recorder.

Lesson 2

(1) Think of something that is:

Red	Grown	In the bathroom
In the sky	Good to eat	Wet
Made of wood	Sharp	Able to fly
Able to swim	In a bedroom	Lovely

(2) Find a word that rhymes with:

Bell	Took
Hate	Moon
Nice	Sun

(3) Read through some letters received by the patient.

(4) Dictation:

'Snow has fallen today and the east wind is very cold. Last year it snowed on the 10th of April!'

(5) Find a word to describe:

A pencil   A tree   A blonde
A man   A house   A film

(6) Answer these questions:

(1) Who is the Pope?

(2) Who is Greta Garbo?

(3) What is snow?

(4) What is wind?

(5) How do you light a fire?

(6) How do you make toast?

(7) Fill in the missing word:

(1) It is cold in here. Please - - - - - the door.

(2) The - - - - - is ringing.

(3) The earth is shaped like a - - - - - .

(4) Where is a piece of - - - - -? I want to write a letter.

(5) I've burnt myself. The coffee is too - - -.

(6) This husband and - - - - - are a good team.

(8) See if the patient can remember the line learnt in the last lesson. ('It is fine today.')

HOMEWORK

Lessons 3 and 4 on the tape recorder. Two more sample lessons are given in Appendix 4.

7 - Include everyday knowledge

All through these lessons we tried to ensure that nothing was omitted in the way of ordinary everyday knowledge.

The Calendar

For instance, can the patient manage the calendar? At the start of each day we asked him to write and say the date, 'Wednesday, April 1st, 1969', or whatever it was, and we checked that he'd got the seasons, months and days in order. We encouraged him to use a diary, to note the weather and the seasonable changes in the country-side, and if he was interested to note the changing night sky.

We continued, to work, too, on mathematical problems, which led to the question of currency.

Money

Can he manage money? You can go through this with him, and even set up a 'pretence' shop where he is the shopkeeper and has to take the money and give the change. Eventually it is good to go shopping with him. Pat came with me to many small local functions where she helped to serve behind 'Bring and Buy' stalls, to run putting competitions, and to officiate at tombolas. This got her out into the world, as it were; made her meet strangers, get used to the confusion of crowds, find stim-ulation, and work at the real thing, however small.

Clocks, Watches and Time

We worked on the clock, discovering that whilst the hands gave the necessary information to the patient the words used to say 'a quarter past twelve', or any other time, were difficult to understand. It is helpful to draw out a big clock face and to write out the words frequently used to express time and also the minutes and hours. Two pencils do as movable hands, or better still two loose bits of cardboard cut as large and small arrows and attached to the centre with a paper fastener. These hands will then swivel round.

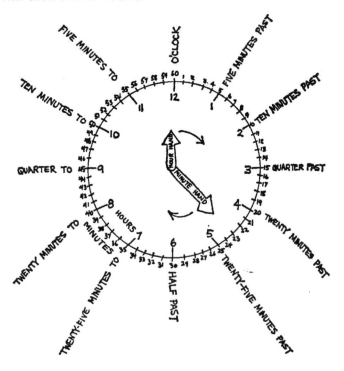

Twenty questions and mime

Using such words or gestures as are at his command, does the patient answer questions accurately? This is particularly important as sometimes questioning by others is the only way he can bring to notice a particular point he wants badly to express. We played a game halfway between Clumps and Twenty Questions. It went like this: The patient thinks of something (say, 'Richard Nixon is President of the United States'). He talks, draws, writes or gestures as best he can to convey what it is. We then ask him question after question. Is it a man? Is he alive? All these questions must only need 'yes' or 'no' as an answer.

Eventually you discover what it is he had in mind. But it is of course essential that he replies 'yes' or 'no' correctly. Doing this as a game prevents him from becoming flustered and confused when people question him in daily conversation, and thus he does not muddle the answers.

Current affairs

Is the patient aware of events that are due to happen, whether they are important current affairs or just going out to dinner that evening? We found it helped to ensure he was up-to-date with everything that was going on, large or small.

Card or board games

Is there any game that he used to play and could try playing again? With both Pat and Alan we found they had played and loved Bridge. This proved wonderful. Look at what you have to do to play Bridge: recognize shapes and colours, sort the cards, count, remember, think for yourself, picture your partner's hand in conjunction with your own, work out a problem, plan ahead, change that plan if necessary, defend a position; a kaleidoscope of brain functions you might well think beyond the powers of a stroke patient.

But look what happened.

As a beginning we discussed it during a lesson, dealt the hands face upwards onto the table, and played them together. One of the teachers made an effective and simple card holder for Alan, whose right hand does not easily cope with the cards. It is a flat piece of wood with two deep grooves cut across it, like this:

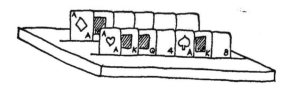

Because neither Pat nor Alan were able at first to say spades, hearts, etc., they used an attractive antique ivory cube on which the suits were marked, like this:

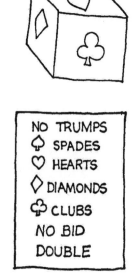

However, you can just as easily draw up a card for the patient to point to if he finds the words hard to say.

Then we started a regular weekly four, learning as we played. Now they both play on equal footing with any of us. They play when they go out to supper, or with anyone whenever a game is going. They steer clear, of course, of the experts, but then so do you and I.

Going places

Can the patient get himself about on his own - use buses, trains or, as a passenger, point out the route to a car driver? He may be understandably nervous of a bus or train journey by himself, so it is perhaps best not to push this. But when he does feel up to such an adventure, it is good to have talked about it with him already. And at his first few attempts you can always supply him with a written list of all the necessary details and information - his own name and address, his destination, type of ticket required etc. - to give him a feeling of security.

As to going in a car as a passenger, we asked him to try to act as guide and map reader. If the journey is long it is worth while studying the route on a map with him beforehand.

All these things are designed to help him take a place in society, and to give him confidence.

8 - A Problem arose

Some strokes seem to wipe out all awareness, to leave the patient inert and apathetic. Pat suffered badly from this, and later, with her great humour and humility, she described her state as that of an enormous pink cabbage. It is frightening at first to meet this inertia, those unfocused eyes and the terrible blankness. You feel as if there is a wall between yourself and the patient, that he does not care a damn about anything, even getting better.

I learned the truth about this by working with Pat, learned the hard way.

If a stroke patient is locked into a windowless cell of inertia there is only one thing he wants to do - get out. He cannot tell you this, and there is a danger of believing the opposite.

When I first went to try to help Pat this inertia hit me squarely between the eyes. It seemed the biggest problem of all. Timorously, I thought I would try a little awakening, something that might act as a stimulant. And to my surprise and joy she reacted with pleasure, made me go on and on until we were both exhausted. She could not have enough of it, and the smallest of sparks appeared in her eyes.

What we did was this. We peppered her with quick unending questions, fired machine gun fashion, from a prepared list, making her answer however best she could, never letting her get away with no reply. I have a pile of foolscap several inches thick closely written on both sides as a memento of this! And indeed you will need thousands of questions if your patient is as insatiable as was Pat. But there is the greatest of rewards in watching the wall of inertia getting chiselled away atom by atom. Any session of questions would go something like this:

(1) Add 7 and 9.

(2) Who is Charles Chaplin?

(3) How old are you?

(4) What is your husband's name?

(5) What day is it?

(6) Who is Hamlet?

(7) Where is Gibraltar?

(8) How do you make a fruit salad?

(9) How are you?

(10) Do you smoke?

(11) Take 21 from 76.

(12) What did you have for breakfast?

(13) Is it raining?

(14) Who is Leonardo da Vinci?

(15) What is the opposite of light?

(16) Where is your home?

(17) Where were you born?

(18) What season is it?

(19) What is the cost of 4 apples at 6p. each?

(20) What colour is butter?

I started with about twenty questions on my list for each lesson and found I needed fifty.

(*There are many sources of lists of questions: books for pub quizes; the game of Trivial Pursuit with different topics are two examples.*)

These questions served another purpose as well as stimulation. They helped to encourage an attempt at speech.

Alan was from the beginning a great deal more aware than Pat - he was left with all his enormous power for hard work, and his great will and determination were not impaired. But his speech was taking longer to return. However, these questions, taken slower, made him struggle with the words to answer them.

Connected to this lack of awareness I found another problem that existed with Pat but not with Alan. During the lessons, as Pat fought to come to life and answer the questions, and as we plied through encyclopedia, dictionary and atlas, it became apparent that she was uncertain of the many facts she had been learning since babyhood. She knew them, and yet had no confidence that what she thought she knew was actually fact. Did the sun really move across the sky each day? Did some trees really shed their leaves every autumn? You can imagine how confusing and destroying such uncertainty must be.

So, again using the reference books, we slowly worked through every single ordinary and tabu subject that we could find. Anything and everything, until her confidence in these facts was restored.

Alan had another almost contrary problem. He has travelled the world, studied, written, noticed and taken part in a thousand things. He is highly intelligent and highly gifted, and as a result has strong opinions with all the consequent wish and need to express them. This was not dulled by his illness. As a result he suffered greatly by having to listen to all of us talking away on all subjects whilst he could not join in. The feeling of frustration must be fearful - and it is certainly something to try to help. We found it important to give him plenty of time to endeavour to express his opinions, and to listen and question him carefully to assist him to get his point across.

With other stroke patients you will perhaps find other worries and, as you spot them, be able to search and work for the best answer you can find.

Another problem we had to overcome was this: as Pat's ability to speak improved, she found that her tiny vocabulary would succeed in getting her point across. Yet the inertia still deadened her will. She did not try to find other, more suitable, words. For instance, 'evil' was the word she found to describe anything that was not perfect. The meal she had eaten was evil, the weather was evil, and a fire that went out was evil.

We had to make a list of these pet words and phrases, and ban them, because, at this stage, although she could probably have found other words, she took the easy way out. It was hindering her progress.

So, much to Pat's fury, we would shrug our shoulders when she said 'evil' for the twentieth time.

'I don't understand you, Pat,' we would say, sitting smugly back in the chair.

'Oh! Oh! Oh! I mean - I mean - I mean EVIL. I mean BAD,' she would answer.

Splendid.

Here are two examples of lessons we gave on the quick fire principle:

Lesson 1
Answer these questions as quickly as you can:
What is your husband's name?

What is his profession?

Where is he now?

What did you have for breakfast?

Where does tea come from?

What is the opposite of black?

Give a word that rhymes with BELL.

What is ice?

Who is Bing Crosby?

Where is Iceland?

What noise does a dog make?

Where does wool come from?

When is Christmas day?

How many inches in a foot?

What is the opposite of HARD?

Who was F. D. Roosevelt?

Give a word that rhymes with TRY.

What is the name of this house?

Multiply 2 X 11.

Do you take sugar in coffee?

When is your birthday?

Who is Micky Mouse?

What is meant by 'ONLY MONKEYS CHATTER'?

(At this halfway stage we had a short breather, and asked the patient to try to memorize the last three words 'Only monkeys chatter'.)

Where is San Francisco?

Who is Shakespeare?

What nationality was Hitler?

What is your home address?

Multiply 5 by what to get a total of 25?

What did you wear yesterday?

A Stroke in the Family

What is my name?

What size shoes do you wear?

What is your telephone number?

Give two girl's names.

What noise does a pig make?

What is the opposite of hot?

What is the capital of France?

Which ocean is the largest?

Complete this line: 'Jack and Jill went up the   .'

How do you light your cigarette?

Add 10 and 14, then take away 3.

What colour is this pencil?

Give two boy's names.

What is this table made of?

How do you spell 'window'?

What day is it?

Mix black and white and what colour results?

See whether the patient can remember the saying learned in this lesson. ('Only monkeys chatter.')

HOMEWORK

Write down 12 towns, 6 rivers, 3 trees, 6 countries, and the names of all your teachers. (Without looking anything up.)

Lesson 2

(Much more difficult. Given to Pat as her ability to speak improved, but her vocabulary was extremely limited.)

(1) Give another word that means the same as:

Stupid	Frequent	Thin	Right
Chair	Neat	Jump	Jersey
Miserable	Yell	Story	Beautiful

(2) Complete the following:

As stiff as -.   As bright as -.

As like as -.   As high as -.

As fat as -.   As green as -.

As brave as -.   As hard as -.

As hot as -.   As pretty as -.

(3) What do these words mean:

Haggard   Humble   Nice

Forgive   Ideal   Thick

Urgent   Confuse   Afraid

(4) Tell me all you know about:

President Lincoln   Winston Churchill

(5) What is the difference between:

A photograph and a painting

Blotting and drawing paper

Evergreen and deciduous trees

Pink and red

Skirt and trousers

Lion and tiger

(6) Name:

6 colours   3 books   3 insects

(7) Say in your own words the meaning of:

To talk shop

A busman's holiday

Once in a blue moon

To pour oil on troubled waters

No smoke without fire

A miss is as good as a mile

HOMEWORK: Write all you can about a circus.

Two more sample lessons are given in Appendix 5

9 - Approaching their former lives

As the patient began to get better we continued to do many of the things outlined in these chapters, but we raised the standard. According to his growing abilities, so we made each subject correspondingly more difficult. However, we also bore strictly in mind this fact: any lesson that proves too hard is a lesson wasted, and will do more harm than good.

After about a year or eighteen months we added to the lessons many different exercises that emphasized speech, memory and imagination.

We asked the patient to read a paragraph, a page from a book or a newspaper column, then made him explain to us what he had just read.

We made him describe things; say, a church, or a football match. Or gave him a picture to study, then asked him to convert it into a word picture, as if describing it to a blind man.

We asked him to tell us all he knew about the Vatican, Walt Disney, Mars, a squirrel, and so on. Then this could be followed up by a discussion and possibly a final checkup in the encyclopedia.

We gave him a list of words, say:

Cowboy	Hot	Saloon
Horse	Gun	Red Indians
Beautiful	Bad	Shot

and asked him to invent a story that included all these words.

When we had both seen a particular play, T.V. programme or film we got him to repeat the story, then discussed it together.

We gave him sentences to learn at the start of a lesson, then asked him to repeat them from memory at the end of the lesson or even next day. And we asked him about something we had done in a lesson a week or a fortnight before.

Or, perhaps most important of all, we just talked together. This gave him an opportunity to bring up any subject under the sun - and we believe you will find there will be many things he wants particularly to discuss.

All this gives you a chance to ensure he has come to terms with himself and his powers, for the more he can express himself the more he can endeavour to work off any nagging fears. It is good, too, that he begins to realize how his efforts can inspire and encourage others.

Return to his old life

There is something else that has not been mentioned so far, yet is important: the question of a stroke patient beginning to take some responsibility again. It must be wise to start this slowly, bit by bit as he improves in capabilities and morale. To push for this too early will promote the wrong sort of stress, but to leave it until too late makes it more difficult and can hinder his recovery. As always, it will be for the partner, in my case Roald Dahl or Lucy Moorehead, to advise how and when it is best to start.

And this brings us to the allied question of how and when does the patient make his first efforts to return to his old life.

Pat's first public appearance

In Pat's case there were two great hurdles to be crossed. She had to face an audience again and she had to learn lines so that her superb gifts as an actress would not be wasted. Only by overcoming these two obstacles could she prove to herself and to everyone else that she had recovered. Not until she had tried would she or anyone else really know. There was no chance of a 'trial'; it had to be a plunge into the deep end.

Some two and a half years after Pat was stricken Roald thought that the time had come to meet the first of these hurdles. He chose something that would help others as well as his wife.

The New York Association for Brain Injured Children asked if Pat would be their guest of honour at a fund raising dinner, and give a speech. Roald accepted. He said that he was not going to accompany her himself as it was important she did this on her own. Instead, he asked me to go along with her, and to speak a few words to introduce Pat at the dinner.

Now Pat and I were in the same boat, a very uncomfortable one, and this, as Roald so wisely knew, was good psychology. We must work at it together - and we were both afraid. Roald and a friend, Barry Farrell, composed the speech, with suggestions from Pat and me. And we set about studying it. We even had a small rehearsal in my home before our friends.

Then, one cold day, off Pat and I went to New York. Could Pat manage a seething mass of press men? Cameras, television, a battery of questions? Until she had tried, no one knew.

A Stroke in the Family

Her New York friends helped to filter the press men into our Waldorf suite six at a time, until the place was crammed. She managed magnificently, visibly gaining in confidence as the six by six entered. Could she stand alone on the stage in the glaring lights and deliver her speech, facing 1,400 people, many of them brain specialists, film stars and friends? Until she had tried, no one knew; not even Pat herself. Again she managed magnificently.

This was a great turning point. Her hopes were high, and there remained only the making of a film. Roald accepted an offer for Pat to star in *The Subject was Roses*. He used the same formula as with the speech. He himself would not go, as she had to do this on her own, and in any case he had job and family to manage. The script was sent over to us in Great Missenden, and we worked and worked at learning it. There were a great many words. By dividing it up into manageable proportions. Pat gradually became familiar with it.

Then, almost a year later, Pat and I again set out for New York, again with our hearts in our mouths. Could she manage it? Again she did - magnificently. The whole company of *The Subject was Roses* were wonderfully kind and helpful. When we returned three months later, on exactly the scheduled date, all Pat's family was there at the airport to cheer.

Every mountain had been climbed.

This chapter, dealing with the last stages of recovery, has referred only to Pat.

9 - Approaching their former lives

Alan's progress

Pat was thirty nine when she was stricken. Alan was in his late fifties. So although the younger the patient, the greater his chance of a good recovery, an age of sixty or even seventy is nothing to be despondent about.

Alan did not start working with the Missenden team until about two years after his illness. He is still working like mad: or going on and on and on, as Alan himself would say. And he is still climbing.

His speech and writing are still very limited. If he wants to say any particular word at any particular time he may not be able to. Alan has asked me to stress this fact, so that no false hopes should be raised. He has been 'at school' for some time now, yet he has not been able actually to learn, as a child can, the easy use of a word he has been taught. What he has achieved in the realm of words is this: he has built up an 'instinctive' vocabulary of words, phrases and sentences which he can say quite normally. This is growing month by month. It has now reached the stage when those who meet him for the first time, and exchange with him the usual little politenesses, do not realize his handicap.

Any effort to improve his speech must come at this 'instinctive' level, where a word gradually filters in like a thief in the night. He can now read aloud provided someone reads with him. His ability to understand the spoken word is fairly good, although it becomes less good when he is faced with a crowd of chattering people. He can read short passages with quick comprehension. Any long or badly written articles he has to study further.

There are other fields, too, where his improvement is marked. He has lost many of the inhibitions of his illness and is more interested in all that goes on around him. He can face crowds, and knows what is going on: in fact, his awareness improves daily. His sense of humour is ever present, and he can now laugh even at himself. There is no doubt that he is wonderfully adjusted to his present limitations.

He is a man with a handicap, not something less than a man.

Here is an example of a lesson given to Pat just before we began studying her speech:

Lesson 1

(1) Learn by heart:

When travelling abroad by air you need your ticket and your passport. You may well also need a vaccination certificate.

(2) Read a newspaper column, and explain its meaning.

(The article for her to read was about the Israel of today.)

(3) What do you know about:

The South Pole

Gypsies

Space exploration

(4) Here are 8 words. Invent a story that includes all of them.

Orchestra Coffee Words Long

Greasepaint Theatre Audience Curtain

(5) Describe:

A garden. Times Square. A magnet.

(6) Tell the story of the play Mame. (Then discuss it and ask questions on points of observation.)

(7) General conversation - here, and throughout the lesson.

(8) Repeat from memory the paragraph learned at the start of the lesson.

HOMEWORK
(Extract from *Everything in the Garden*, by Giles Cooper)
Learn Jenny's part.

BERNARD: Where did you get five hundred pounds?

JENNY : *I didn't steal it.*

BERNARD: Where did you get it?

JENNY: *I earned it.*

BERNARD: A job, you've got a job.

JENNY: *Sort of.*

BERNARD : I said I didn't want you to take a job. Anyway you couldn't have, not this sort of job. ... I mean five hundred pounds, you couldn't have had it long anyway.

JENNY: *Six weeks.*

BERNARD: No look, darling, look. Tell me. Did someone leave it to you? Did someone die and you haven't told me?

JENNY: *Nobody died. I earned it. In the afternoons.*

BERNARD: Even if you worked full time you couldn't have earned this sort of money. Oh no. Come on now. Tell me.

JENNY : *I make twenty five guineas five afternoons, a week, sometimes more. I spent a little on clothes but there hasn't been time to spend the rest.*

BERNARD: Nobody pays that sort of money, and I

mean you've no training.

JENNY : *You don't need any.*

BERNARD: What do you need?

JENNY: *Your coffee's still warm, or shall I heat it up?*

A few more ideas for these final lessons are given in Appendix 6.

Editor's Note:

Clearly, as a performer, Pat's goal was easily defined. It was not so easy for Alan, nor I suspect will it be easy for the readers. In my case as a member of a self-help group, I can imagine several ways in which a patient can set a realistic goal with the help of friends and other members of the group. For example, such a group has a number of jobs that need to be done: membership records; organizing outings; collecting and paying for a group lunch or tea. At some gatherings, it is necessary to propose thanks: to a host or speaker; for the special efforts of a member, for example.

But you do not have to belong to a group to get similar benefits. A family visit to the local takeaway requires some organization; who wants what; who pays; have you got the right money; or do you get the correct change.

Engage your patient in these and similar activities to bring up his self-esteem – provided you are confident that they will be within his power. Planning with him was the key for Pat, as it will be for you.

10 - Acknowledgments

What has been written here is an accumulation of ideas built up from all Pat and Alan's friends-turned-teachers. You will have many new ideas of your own, particularly bearing in mind that every stroke patient will have different problems. It is part of the merit of Roald's system that each teacher contributes his own skills and uses his own imagination to gain his objective.

There is no phoney sob-stuff about this being rewarding work. It is rewarding work.

Lastly, and by far the most important, none of this would have got off the ground without humanity and courage.

It is the human understanding of one man, Roald Dahl, which led to the whole idea.

And it is owing to the really great courage of Patricia Neal and Alan Moorehead, and no less of Roald Dahl and Lucy Moorehead, that any progress was made at all.

A Stroke in the Family

Acknowledgments

The Team for Patricia Neal	*The Team for Alan Moorehead*
ELSE LOGSDAIL	ROALD DAHL
ALFHILD HANSEN	ELSE LOGSDAIL
ASTA ANDERSON	ALFHILD HANSEN
MARJORIE CLIPSTONE	PATRICIA KIRWAN DICK
PATRICIA KIRWAN	KIRWAN MARJORIE
ANGELA KIRWAN	CLIPSTONE MARGOT
JOAN HENLEY	HORNBY RITA DUFF
JANE FIGG	LAWRENCE DUFF
JUDY KNYVETTE-HOFF	VALERIE EATON
PEGGY NEWLAND	GRIFFITH
VALERIE EATON	
GRIFFITH	

Reserves	Reserves
FRANKIE CONQUY	ASTA ANDERSON
JEAN MORGAN	JUDY KNYVETTE-HOFF
	TESSA DAHL

The once-a-week Bridge Team for Pat and Alan

DAPHNE EATON GRIFFITH	ELIZABETH FULTON
JO ROBINSON	PATRICIA NEAL
EATON GRIFFITH	(working with Alan
AUDREY RAE SMITH	Moorehead)
PATRICIA KIRWAN	VALERIE EATON GRIFFITH

Appendix 1

Here are two more lessons approximately the same standard as those given in Chapter 3.

Lesson 1

(1) Go through the general idea that is involved in the game of Snap. Then start to play like this :

With a pack of cards each, both of you turn the cards face upwards one by one in unison. When the card turned up by one player exactly matches the card turned up by the other, get the patient to say 'snap' as soon as he sees the identical cards. If he cannot say the word 'snap', get him to shout out. From time to time chivy him up by yelling 'snap' yourself.

When he's got the idea, play a proper game with him. (It is possible to increase the number of times when both players turn up the same card by using only the spades and hearts from 4 packs.)

(2) Show him a tray on which are 4 objects: say, a box of matches, a pencil, a watch and a spoon. Let him study it for a while. Then remove the tray from his sight, take something away, and return the tray now laden with 3 objects to him. Can he communicate to you what is missing? Repeat this, taking a different object off each time and speeding up the whole process.

(3) Give the patient a paint brush, a jar of water and a box of water colours containing only the primaries and black and white.

First, get him to point to the colours as you call them

out. Then ask him to mix two colours together in the palette so that the resultant colour is:

Green   Cream
Grey   Pink
Orange   Brown
Purple   Navy blue

(4)   Ask the patient to communicate to you the difference between:

A tree and a bush
A house and a flat
The STOP and GO of traffic lights
A canary and a blackbird
Sunset and dawn
A cup and a mug

(d) What is missing in the following?

(1) AA   + +   B.   .
(2) 26.36.46.56.66.   . 86.96.
(3) 4 + 6 +   + 2 = 15.

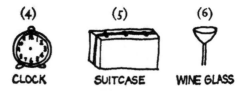

(4)   (5)   (6)
CLOCK   SUITCASE   WINE GLASS

(6) Play clock golf on the carpet. Using a putter, a golf ball and a ring of numbers placed around a box turned on its side, putt out the course in as few strokes as possible.

HOMEWORK
Sort a shuffled pack of cards into suits and put each suit into numerical order.

Lesson 2

(1) Open an atlas at a map of the world. Ask the patient to point out:

United States	Australia
Great Britain	Pacific Ocean
North Pole	Japan
France	Equator

Move on to towns, mountains, and rivers if he is managing this well.

(2) Sketch a few national flags in colour and ask the patient to point to each relevant country.

(3) Close the atlas and see whether he can open it at a map of Scotland, Canada, Germany. Can he find his own home town and point to the hills, rivers, lakes etc. that make up its natural setting?

(4) Hide your own efforts at drawing the flags and see whether the patient can reproduce them.

(5) Which is the odd-man-out in the following?

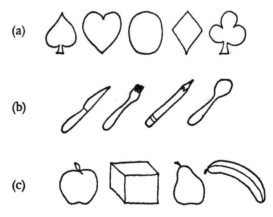

(6) Making sure these things are in the room where you are working, ask the patient to point to the following:

Ask these questions after he has communicated to you

the answers to the first question

(a) TOES

How many have you?

What colour are they?

(b) WOOL

What is its natural colour?

Where does it grow?

What use has it?

(C) WINE

What fruit produces it?

In which countries does the fruit grow ?

What is its effect on people?

(d) WOOD

Where does it come from?

Is there more than one sort?

What creatures may live in these trees?

(7) Work together on a game of patience (e.g. clock patience) to enable the patient to play it when he is on his own.

(8) (a) Ask the patient to take the matches out of a match box and to count them, perhaps in groups of ten.

(b) Ask him to take twelve away and tell you how many are left.

(c) Using as many matches as he likes, ask him to make a square, a rectangle, a diamond, a half-circle, the letter H, a five-bar gate.

(It is interesting to note that Alan drew the letter H correctly, along with most of the other shapes. Yet when asked to write it in connection with the alphabet he could not.)

HOMEWORK

Give him a list of objects to learn and remember for the next lesson. For example :

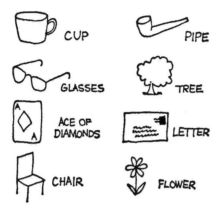

Appendix 2

Here are two more lessons of approximately the same standard as those given in Chapter 4. But these lessons also include a simple start to some of the general material from Chapter 7.

Lesson 1

(1) Choose a very short piece from the newspaper. (It is best to select a subject that is either of particular interest to the patient or a talking-point of the moment.)

Read it with him several times, then ask him to communicate to you what it was about.

(2) In simple terms start working on the calendar.

Check the seasons through carefully with him, making sure the transition through spring, summer, autumn and winter is fully understood.

Using a calendar with a seasonal picture for each month, begin working through the full twelve months.

Set out the seven days of the week and discuss which days are working ones and which weekend.

Check that he appreciates the meaning of today, tomorrow, yesterday, this year, last month, next week, ten years ago etc.

With the calendar in front of him, ask him today's date. Then get him to write it out.

(3) Find the correct sentence by unmixing these words:
MET NMA ESGO OT KWRO YB RCA
and again with these words:
LUJY SI A YVER MWRA HMTON

(4) Play a mixture of Clumps and Twenty Questions with the patient. (One of the most difficult problems at this stage is to gain his interest. Therefore it is vital to lose no chance of this simply because the patient cannot communicate it to you. Maybe there will be some subjects that he would like information on: perhaps the progress of a friend or an international situation.)

Ask him to think up something he would like to hear about. When he has thought of something ask him to try to illustrate it with pencil and paper and with gestures. As he draws and gestures you ask him question after question. Each of these questions is phrased so that it only needs a 'Yes' or 'No', nod or shake of the head. Eventually the answer is discovered. You then talk about it as best you can. If it is a subject you know little or nothing about, it is well worth while finding out and discussing it at the next lesson.

HOMEWORK
(1) Think up some further subjects for Clumps/Twenty Questions.
(2) Write out the seasons, months and days of the week.

Lesson 2

(1) Turn on the television or radio when a short news programme is being broadcast. Listen to it with the patient, then see if he can communicate to you any of the subject matter. Discuss it with him.
(2) Give him a clock face, with movable hands, that you have made before the lesson. See whether he can use it to answer these questions:

   (a) When do you get up in the mornings?

(b) When do you have breakfast?

(c) When do you have lunch?

(d) When do you have supper?

(e) When do you go to bed?

(f) When do you have your lessons?

(g) What time is it now?

According to how he manages this, go through with him the problems of telling the time.

(3) Make as many words as possible using only these letters:

(a) PSNIE   (b) TRAHTEE

Ask the patient to pick out the rhyming words when he has completed each list.

(4) Ask him the following questions (if necessary, using the calendar):

(a) What day is it today?

(b) When is it likely to snow?

(c) When is your birthday?

(d) When is Christmas day?

(e) What day will tomorrow be?

(f) When is Easter?

(g) When does spring begin?

(h) What day was yesterday?

(i) Which is the last day of the year?

(5) Talk to the patient about his immediate surroundings, encouraging him to copy your words as each item is observed and mentioned. You can do this in any number of places, but perhaps the easiest are:

In your work room.

Looking out of the window.

Walking up and down a street.

In your garden.

If you begin in the room where you are sitting, the lesson might start like this:

(a) The window is open. (The window is shut.)

(b) The table is made of wood.

(c) The light is on. (The light is off.)

(d) There is a fly on the wall.

(e) The picture is crooked. (I will straighten it.)

and continue on these lines.

Each sentence can be repeated several times (with actions where applicable) and the patient will try saying them with you.

HOMEWORK

(1) Look at a particular television programme with a view to communicating the substance of it to you at the next lesson. (Choose one that the teacher will also have a chance of seeing.)

(2) Start on a jigsaw that is a little harder than the previous one.

Appendix 3

Here are two more lessons approximately at the same standard as those given in Chapter 5. But these lessons also include a simple start to some more of the general material from Chapter 7.

Lesson 1

(1) Uncover a tray on which are four cards, each with a word printed on it. For example: FIRE APPLE BATH MATCH.

Ask the patient to study these words, and to try to remember them.

(2) Testing both his memory and his observation, ask him to answer the following questions:

(a) What did you have for lunch yesterday?

(b) What was I wearing yesterday?

(c) What is the colour of the pencil you are using? (First put your hand over it.)

(d) What is the colour of your bedroom curtains?

(e) What was the weather like yesterday?

(f) What did you do the day before yesterday?

(3) In simple terms start working with money. Lay all the different notes and coins on the table.

Ask the patient to point to each one as you call out its name - 10p, £1, 50p, £5 and so on.

According to how he manages this, tax him further with questions such as:

(a) You want to buy a newspaper costing sixty pence. Will you give me the money for it?

(b) You want to buy two newspapers costing sixpence each. Will you give me the money for them?

(c) You want to buy a box of chocolates costing £1.40p. Will you give me the money for it?

(d) You want to buy five apples at ten pence each. How much will it cost you?

Make sure the patient understands the way of writing money, e.g. £2.15p.

(4) What is wrong with the following:

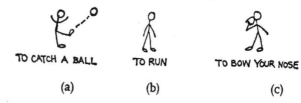

TO CATCH A BALL	TO RUN	TO BOW YOUR NOSE
(a)	(b)	(c)

(d) There are no shadows when the sun is out.

(e) The equator encircles the earth, passing through the North and South Poles.

(f) The last Great War lasted from 1936 to 1945.

(5) See whether the patient can remember the four words he studied at the start of the lesson. Ask him to draw and write them.

HOMEWORK

(1) What is the cost of 4 books at £2.50p. each?

(2) What is the cost of 3 postcards at 12p. each?

(3) What is the cost of 7 pens at 16p. each?

(4) What is the cost of one toy at £3.75p. and a packet of notepaper at 75p.?

(5) What is 65p. less 24p.?

(6) Add £1 43p., 53p. and 4p.?

(7) Collect a small pile of money and count it.

Lesson 2

At this stage we found it wise to check on the patient's ability to understand and cope with many other everyday things.

A lesson can be used profitably in discovering what he can manage in each of these fields and where he needs help.

TELEPHONE
(1) See if he can dial the number of a friend.
(2) Can he understand the person talking at the other end?
(3) Can he manage to say a few words to them?

It is an interesting fact that Alan found he talked his best on the phone. We used a second house telephone during some lessons and carried on a pupil/teacher conversation, each of us sitting alone in a room. It may well be worth while to try this with other stroke patients.

STAMPS
At some time when you have an assorted collection of letters to go to the post, see whether the patient can stick the correct stamp on each one.

CHEQUES
(1) Does he understand the point of writing a cheque?
(2) If you make out a dummy cheque can he fill it in?
(3) Using a bank balance and cheques, instead of cash, does he understand the currency?

WEIGHTS AND MEASURES
Can he cope with these as encountered in ordinary life? For instance:

(1) Can he evaluate how many pints of milk are needed each day, and move the milk-dial to the amount required for tomorrow?

(2) If you have a temperature gauge inside or outside your home, can he read and understand it?

(3) Can he make a fair guess at the number of miles apart one place is from another? If he does not know the answer, can he find it out from a map?

THE SKY

(1) Can he point to north, south, east and west?

(2) Can he tell you where the wind is coming from?

(3) Can he tell you which side of a tree the shadow would fall were the sun out at any given time?

(4) Can he tell you where the sun will rise and set?

(5) Can he tell you why the moon varies from full to crescent?

(6) Can he tell you which is the sunny quarter in the Southern Hemisphere?

As you work together you will probably find more of these everyday things about which the patient is uncertain. As soon as you make each small discovery, it is important to get to work on it quickly. The lack of this 'taken-for-granted' knowledge greatly increases the patient's feeling of being an outcast in an alien world.

HOMEWORK

A crossword that includes some of the material from this lesson.

Appendix 4

Here are two more lessons of approximately the same standard as those given in Chapter 6.

Lesson 1

(1) Read together and discuss the following sentence:
    'Two new houses have been built in our road.'
Make sure the patient has built up a word picture of it, then ask him to memorize it.

(2) Think of a word that has the opposite meaning to:

Cold	Hard	Small
Wet	Tall	Empty
Above	Dark	Up
Nice	On	Good

(3) Give the patient a coloured picture to study. Say, a busy town crossroad on a sunny day. With the picture in front of him, ask him the following questions:

(a) Where is north?

(b) Do you think the picture was taken on a weekday or during the week-end? Why?

(c) How many pedestrians are visible?

(d) What shops can you see?

(e) Approximately what is the temperature of the day?

(f) What change will there be in this scene by midnight?

Now take the picture away and ask him these questions :

(a) Is there a taxi in the picture?

(b) What colour are the cars?

(c) Are the traffic lights at 'Stop' or 'Go'?

(d) Is the sun out?

(e) Is there a policeman in the picture?

(f) What signposts are visible?

(4) Find the correct sentence by unmixing and putting in order these words:

pselpa rlaye oD ntuAmu? hte ipnre ni

(5) Think of:

(a) Four things you like to eat.

(b) Four things you like to drink.

(c) Three implements you use to eat with.

(d) Two containers you use to drink from.

(6) Can the patient remember the sentence he learned at the start of the lesson?

HOMEWORK

Give the patient four groups of words to unmix and assemble into four sentences (as in No. 4 of this lesson).

Lesson 2

(1) Make up sentences using these words:

(a) Car. Driver. Wheel.

(b) Table. Chair. Typewriter.

(c) Garden. Flower. Red. Earth.

(2) Think of a word that means the same as:

Breeze	Plump	Scarlet
Pretty	Light	Large
Healthy	Human being	Level

Look up each one in the dictionary after the patient has tried to find his own word.

(3) Mimic the sound made by each of the following:

Sheep	Fog horn	Horse	Telephone engaged signal
Bell	Owl	Dog	Bee
Cow	Clock	Cat	Train

(4) Pick out the matching pairs in the following group of words:

Knife	Red	Bread	Clubs
Mortar	Spades	Pen	Bricks
Butter	Fork	Paper	Black

(5) Complete the following sentences:

   (a) People grow roses because...

   (b) I hate the cold weather because ...

   (c) He ate a great deal because ...

   (d) David and Jane have a large car because ...

   (e) The film was a success because...

   (f) The paper was peeling off the walls because ...

HOMEWORK

Give the patient an article from the newspaper to read and study. Warn him that you will be discussing this with him at the next lesson.

Appendix 5

Here are two more lessons of approximately the same standard as those given in Chapter 8.

Lesson 1

(1) Give the patient a 1 inch to the mile local map. Tell him that, in ten minutes or so, you are both going to drive to a chosen place and he is going to direct you there.

Where and how far you go must of course depend on where you start from. Living in Great Missenden, our lesson went like this:

(a) Plan a route to Marlow bridge.

(b) Get in the car and ask him to direct you to this destination, sticking to the chosen route. (The patient can use the map as he goes along if necessary, or direct you from memory. He must say 'right', 'left' or 'straight on' at every turning.)

(c) On arrival we met a friend for coffee. This had been arranged beforehand, and the patient was encouraged to take his part in the conversation.

(d) On the return journey he is relieved of his responsibilities as guide. Instead you pepper him with questions such as:

(1) How long does this journey take us?

(2) Why am I braking?

(3) What gear am I in?

(4) How fast am I driving?

(5) What is that shop selling?

(6) How old is that woman going across the road?

(7) What make is the car ahead?

(8) What is the number of the car ahead?

(9) How do I know when the car ahead is braking?

(10) What is being built ahead of us?

(11) What is that lorry carrying?

(12) What is written on that notice?

(13) Are we in a 30 m.p.h. limit?

(14) About how far are we from Marlow now?

(15) What is the name of the friend we met for coffee?

(16) Did she take sugar in her coffee?

(17) Did she smoke?

(18) What does that sign '1 in 6' mean?

(19) Where does that turning go to?

(20) How near home are we?

HOMEWORK

From memory, draw a map of our route to Marlow.

Lesson 2

(1) Choose carefully a list of words and phrases that the patient uses too often and sometimes inaccurately. Ask him to substitute something else on each of the following occasions :

(a) Evil

The weather is evil. The weather is -.

The film was evil. The film was -.

The wine was evil (meaning too sweet).

The wine was -

My shoe is evil (meaning too tight). My shoe is -.

(b) Marvellous

The play was marvellous. The play was -.

The soup was marvellous. The soup was -.

Mary is marvellous (meaning I like Mary).

Mary is -.

The dress is marvellous (meaning pretty).

The dress is -

(c) Larger and larger

The tree is getting larger and larger. The tree is -.

Jack is getting larger and larger (meaning fatter). Jack is getting -.

Each week I can read larger and larger (meaning more).

Each week I can read -.

My days are getting larger and larger (meaning busier). My days are -.

(2) Go shopping with the patient.

(a) Have a prepared list of several things you or he will want to buy.

(b) Get him to transact the business on his own. (Preferably visiting the ordinary shops. Post Office and bank.)

(c) Get him to phone home from a public telephone box, working the machine on his own.

HOMEWORK

Type a letter to an imaginary shop ordering all the ingredients needed for a dinner party for six people.

Appendix 6

Here are a few more ideas to help the patient as he embarks on the last stages of his recovery:

Responsibility.
Probably for several years now the patient has been concerned only with his own recovery. He has not been in a position to take responsibility in any other shape or form.

His household will have settled into a routine built on this assumption. And his friends will be firmly in the habit of excluding him from any extra burden. It will not be easy either for the patient or for his immediate associates to change this now well-established custom. But slowly it must be changed.

We began in the following way:

(a) As normal conversation began to occupy about half of each lesson we introduced into it other people's troubles.

The aim was to give the patient a chance to become outward-looking again: increasingly to think of others and to shift the inevitable emphasis from himself.

(b) At home and during the lessons he was asked to perform some small task. Maybe it was only to remember to buy something, to concoct a menu or to deliver a message.

It does not matter how small the matter is. But it does matter that his efforts are not checked upon. If he fails, all right, he fails.

Gradually he will learn to succeed, and gradually we will learn that he can be relied upon. He, too, will begin to realize that we are relying on him.

Outings.

All the way through his recovery outings are important, but at this final stage they are vital.

There are many possibilities here, but the choice must depend primarily on the patient's interests and the accessibility of the venue.

We found the following stood us in good stead:

(a) A day's shopping in London.

(b) A visit to Whipsnade Zoo.

(c) A visit to the Rothschild estate at Waddesdon.

(d) Going to a child's sports-day.

(e) A visit to Blenheim Palace.

(f) Going to a picture gallery to help choose a painting.

(g) A visit to Windsor Castle.

(h) Making his own way by bus or train to meet a friend.

(i) Visits to the theatre or a sporting event.

(j) A visit to the Public Gallery of the House of Commons to listen to a debate.

Return to Work

Finally, there is the possibility of the patient's returning to work.

You will have seen in Chapter 9 how we approached this in Pat's case. Naturally each person is different. But it is wise to make every effort you can to lessen the height of this final hurdle.

Appendix 7

The period that this book covers is the last years of the 1960's. The world then was quite different from today.

Neighbourhoods
Most of us live in towns. Many no longer know their neighbours. Others spend every evening glued to the TV, or to computers attached to the internet where they can blog or play games. Children are discouraged or even forbidden to play outside. Almost all parents are working and have little or no time to spare. So where can you find your volunteers who are to visit your home and give these vital lessons to your patient?

Fortunately there are many organisations who offer volunteer help. The local library will have a noticeboard or list with contact details of many local societies and clubs covering a wide range of interests. Your GP will have contacts, who will have contacts.

The local clubs and societies, whether sporting or leisure may often have members with that vital hour of spare time every week or two. Singers in the area's choir, or muscians will be able to bring an insight into music - aided by examples from their CD collections. Stamps are rich in a variety of topics: geographical, political, historical, and an enthusiast from the local club may be a welcome change for your patient.

Props
The author and her colleagues spent time making many props to aid understanding. The child of today is very-

fortunate to have an entire industry devoted to educating them. Anyone with a young child in the family knows very well that the toy box is full of 'educational toys'. Here is a rich seam of treasures, matching words to pictures, learning how to tell the time, catalogues full of books for the child to learn geography, history, locomotives, sailing. Make a trip to your charity shops, to the library (children's section), and here you will surely find inspiration and practical examples.

The government has introduced strategies for literacy and numeracy. These have provoked enterprises to produce teaching aids specifically for these subjects. A visit to www.yellowmoon.org.uk will retrieve a collection of very suitable material that is far from expensive.

However

It may be that your patient has or grows an intolerance of the obvious childishness of the toys. In that case you may resort to the home made exhibits that our author used.

Caution

Giving an aphasic or disphasic patient mental exercise and stimulus, to assist recovery, requires minds that are clear of hidden agendas or other distractions (problems, worries etc.). It is our experience at East Kent Strokes that spouses or partners of the patient are most often less able to empty their own minds of their joint relationships. And so, the spouse is usually the last person capable of teaching their loved one, their patient. It is virtually impossible to begin a fresh conversation with someone with whom you have lived for years. Whatever the topic, as one speaks the other reacts, and this reaction - a raised eyebrow, sharp intake of breath - can be interpreted in the context of yesterday's argument, last month's disappointment, the tragedy from two years ago.

There is a role for the spouse, and it is amply described here. Roald Dahl had his hands full with running the family and home. Pat had a child just months after her stroke, so you will have an idea of the pressures that Roald faced. As far as the teaching was concerned, he spent his time recruiting volunteers, arranging their timetable, and making sure of the stock of coffee and biscuits - but took no part in the actual lessons - except as a bridge partner.

At EKS, the carers of our speechless members are climbing up the wall with the frustration of having no one to talk to. Their knee jerk answers to their patients' cries of help were often counter-productive. For one couple, he constantly asked "Why?" to which she could only answer "I don't know!". Later, a different member took him under her wing and soon became exasperated with his Why's. He accepted her admonishment and command "No more Why's, or I'm going home". His wife would never have said this because of the love she still bears for him and the fear of just making things worse.

So, if you are the spouse or partner, steel yourself to finding your team of volunteers, and leave them to their task of stimulating your patient's brain. Put a distance between the teaching process and your 'normal' daily living routine. This way lies success.

Appendix 7

Children

Kids have two assets that they can bring to your aid. Firstly, as described in chapter 6, they are uninhibited when talking to the patient. The confidence that this will bring to him cannot be over emphasised. Secondly, they will have internet skills that you may lack. Harness them to find groups who may supply your volunteers, or sources of materials and examples. There really are so many items to be found. (However - be warned that searching for websites with the term 'stroke' can bring the wrong results!).

David Worsley

Some useful contacts

Stroke Association to empower stroke survivors and carers to positively influence policy and the provision of stroke services locally across England. Visit http://www.stroke.org.uk/

Connect is a charity for people living with aphasia, a communication disability which usually occurs after stroke. It can also be caused by brain injury or tumour. Visit http://www.ukconnect.org/

Headway To promote understanding of all aspects of brain injury and to provide information, support and services to people with a brain injury, their families and carers. Visit http://www.headway.org.uk/

Our website contains a list of contacts. Visit www.eastkentstrokes.com